EVERYDAY AIDS AND APPLIANCES

EVERYDAY AIDS AND APPLIANCES

Edited by

GRAHAM P MULLEY, DM, FRCP

*Consultant geriatrician, Department of
Medicine (Elderly), St James's University
Hospital, Leeds*

Articles from the *British Medical Journal*

Published by the British Medical Journal
Tavistock Square, London WC1H 9JR

First published 1989
Second impression 1991

British Library Cataloguing in Publication Data

Everyday aids and appliances
 1. Equipment for physically handicapped
persons
 I. Mulley, Graham P (Graham Peter) II. British
medical journal
 362.4'028

ISBN 0-7279-0241-5

Typesetting by Bedford Typesetters Ltd, Bedford
Printed in Great Britain by Latimer Trend & Co Ltd, Plymouth

Contents

Introduction

Nearly one in 10 of the adult population of England and Wales is disabled. Despite the large number of disabled people who can benefit from aids, and the high cost of provision, far less attention is given to rehabilitation aids than to equipment used for diagnosis and treatment. The use of technical aids can enable a disabled person to do more for himself and therefore feel better; they can also make caring easier. The word "aids" is used here to include those items of equipment which compensate for decline in or loss of function. In the series of articles republished in this book the authors consider aids that are attached to the body (hearing aids, stomas, collars and corsets, pads and pants, catheters, special footwear, stockings, artificial legs); those held by but not necessarily fixed to the body (mobility aids, low visual aids, certain communication aids); equipment in the home which allows independence in everyday activities (bath and toilet aids, wheelchairs, easy chairs, hoists); the function of disabled living centres; and how the provision of aids and appliances can be improved.

Disability is most prevalent in the elderly. Two thirds of the very seriously handicapped are over 75. Eighty per cent of visually disabled people are of retirement age, half being over 75. Only 64% of the elderly are fully independent in bathing and over half the women over 85 living at home need aids or help to get to and from the toilet. Thus emphasis is given to the relatively simple aids required for the elderly disabled; but some of the more sophisticated aids required by the younger handicapped person are also considered.

An awareness of the range of items available allows clinicians to ensure that their disabled patients obtain appropriate and useful aids. It will also equip them to determine whether an aid is acceptable and safe. Aids and appliances can be recommended with confidence only if the doctor is convinced of their efficacy. As well as outlining which aids are available and describing how to obtain them the authors also critically evaluate evidence for their effectiveness. I hope that this book will promote a greater interest in those everyday aids which can make such a difference to the lives of disabled people and their families.

GRAHAM P MULLEY

Hearing aids

OLIVER J CORRADO

Deafness is a common problem which increases in prevalence with age, 60% of people over 70 having some degree of hearing loss. There are two types of hearing loss: conductive, caused by lesions which interfere with the transmission of sound anywhere from the exterior to the end of the ossicular chain; and sensorineural, caused by lesions of the cochlea or auditory nerve. Hearing aids should be considered for patients with impaired hearing when definitive treatment is complete or when it is impossible. They act by amplifying incoming sound so that it is heard at a more effective level.[1]

Obtaining an aid

Twenty per cent of hearing aids are not used within six months of being supplied, so before referring adult patients it is worth ensuring that hearing loss is affecting their lifestyle and that they are prepared to wear an aid once it is supplied. An aid should be considered for any child whose deafness is impeding natural speech development.[2] To obtain a National Health Service hearing aid a patient must be referred to an ear, nose, and throat consultant, who will assess the patient and arrange a pure tone audiogram. If the patient is a suitable candidate for a hearing aid an ear mould impression will be taken and an aid supplied later. Aids with temporary earpieces may be supplied in the interim. The whole process can take a long time; but many health authorities implement direct referral to hearing aid clinics, thus reducing delay.

Types of aid

The choice of aid for a particular patient depends on age, the amount of amplification required, the ability to manage the controls, and the presence of other aural disease—for example, otorrhoea.[3]

1

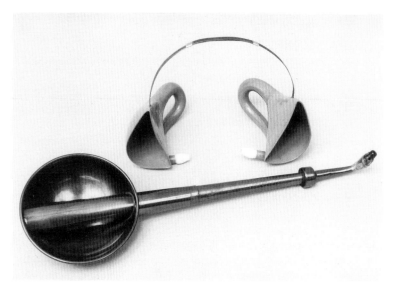

Head worn *(above)* and metal hand held *(below)* ear trumpets. Both these models are now obsolete.

Non-electric hearing aids can still be obtained through the National Health Service. Two types are available: telescopic and non-telescopic plastic ear trumpets. Although outdated they are still used for the occasional elderly patient who has difficulty using an electronic aid. Of the electronic aids, those carried within the ear are the most discreet, but they are available only in special circumstances. They are useful for people who also have to wear protective headwear (such as helmets); however, as their ability to amplify sound is limited they are unsuitable for patients with severe hearing loss.

The commonest types of electronic hearing aids readily available on the National Health Service are postaural aids (BE or "behind ear" aids) and body worn aids (BW aids).

Postaural aids are the most widely used. Three ranges are available. These differ according to the amount of gain they can provide and so are suitable for different degrees of hearing loss. The BE10 series (BE11-17) is suitable for mild to moderate hearing impairment, the BE30 series (BE31-35) for moderate hearing impairment, and the BE50 series (BE51-53) for more profound hearing loss.

In postaural aids speech and environmental sounds are picked up by the microphone, which is generally situated at the base or facing forwards at the top of the aid. The case contains the amplifier,

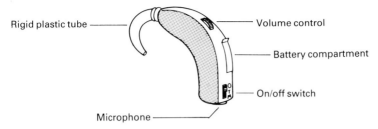

Rigid plastic tube — Volume control

— Battery compartment

— On/off switch

Microphone —

Postaural (BE) aid.

receiver, and battery compartment. A mercury camera battery is standard, although zinc–air batteries, which last nearly twice as long, can be used for aids of the BE10 and 30 series. All aids have a volume control which can be operated by the user and a switch with settings marked O for the off position, M for the on (microphone) position, and T, which is for use with telephones fitted with an inductive coupler (telecoil) and which cuts out background noise. All public telephones are fitted with these. They can be fitted into most private telephones by British Telecom at a cost of £13.80 (including value added tax); financial help, if required, can often be obtained from local authorities. (British Telecom has a large range of equipment suitable for the hard of hearing.) Some public buildings (churches, theatres, conference halls, etc) are also fitted with a loop system enabling aid wearers to use the pick up coil.

Causes of conductive deafness

Congenital
Deformity of the pinna
Meatal stenosis or atresia
Congenital cholesteatoma
Ossicular fixation
Association with many
  congenital defects

Acquired
Wax
Foreign bodies
Inflammatory meatal stenosis
Tumours of auditory canal
  or middle ear

Perforation or scarring of ear
  drum
Middle ear effusion
Acute otitis media
Chronic otitis media
Secretory otitis media
  (glue ear)
Traumatic rupture of
  ossicles
Barotrauma
Otosclerosis
Paget's disease
Eustachian tube dysfunction

Causes of sensorineural deafness

Congenital and neonatal
Genetic
Maternal infections, eg rubella,
  syphilis, measles,
  toxoplasmosis, and
  cytomegalovirus
Perinatal complications,
  eg hypoxia and
  hyperbilirubinaemia
Neonatal infections,
  eg meningitis and encephalitis

Acquired
Viral infections, eg mumps
  and measles

Bacterial infections,
  eg meningitis
Trauma, eg head injury and
  skull fracture
Noise and blast injury
Oval or round window rupture
Menière's disease
Labyrinthitis due to chronic
  middle ear disease
Syphilis
Metabolic disorders
Presbycusis
Multiple sclerosis
Drugs, eg aminoglycosides
Tumours, eg acoustic neuroma

Ear moulds are generally made of acrylic plastic but can be made from materials that are not allergenic. They can be either soft or hard, and different colours are available to suit varying skin tones and pigmentation. The ear mould should fit snugly into the outer ear and extend for 5–10 mm into the auditory canal to relay sound to the drum. Open moulds (so called because they have a central hole enabling sound to reach the drum directly) may be more acceptable to the patient and help reduce background noise; a similar effect can be obtained by drilling a small hole ("vent") in the mould.[4] Postaural aids will usually fit comfortably even when worn with spectacles, but if necessary the spectacle side arm can be modified to incorporate a hearing aid adapter.

Patients who have difficulty in managing the controls of a postaural aid should be considered for a body worn aid. The BW61 and BW81 aids can provide a greater amount of gain than postaural aids and so are useful for patients with severe hearing loss. (The Medresco OL aids—so called because they were designed to meet Medical Research Council otolaryngological specifications—have been superseded by the newer electronic aids; the only model still available is the OL56, which is soon to be withdrawn.) Body worn aids have a volume control which can be operated by the user. It is combined with the on/off switch in the BW81 aid but is separate in the BW61 aid. Both BW61 and BW81 aids have T and MT switch positions, the latter enabling

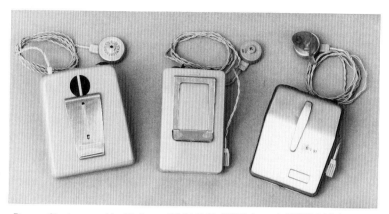

Range of body worn aids: Medresco OL56 *(left)*, BW61 *(centre)*, BW81 *(right)*.

microphone and telecoil to be used simultaneously. The BW61 also has a separate tone control marked N for normal and H for high. The H position is useful to cut out low tone sounds when there is a lot of background noise. The earphone for body worn aids is connected to the aid by a cord and is fitted directly to the ear mould. BW61 and BW81 aids can be used as bone conductors, a vibrator held in place with a headband replacing the earphone. Bone conductors are used for patients who have middle ear disease associated with chronic otorrhoea. Body worn aids use a simple pen battery and have a clip to secure the aid to clothing. Small purses to hold these aids can be obtained from the Royal National Institute for the Deaf. Severely deaf children should be fitted with two (binaural) aids, since speech development depends on good hearing.[2]

Care of the aid

Patients should be advised on how to care for their aid.[5] Batteries should be stored in a cool, dry place and spares should be kept (particularly when the patient is going on holiday). Batteries can last from a few days to several weeks, depending on the type of battery, power of the aid, use, and volume setting. New batteries can be obtained from hearing aid centres or health centres, and used mercury batteries should be returned so that the mercury can be recycled. The aid should be kept out of direct sunlight and removed for bathing or going to the hairdresser. Hair spray tends to clog up the aid and should either not be used or be applied before fitting the aid. The ear

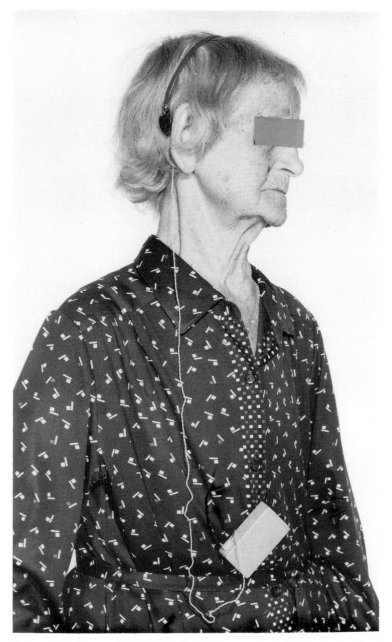

Patient with body worn aid (BW61) fitted with a bone conductor held in place by a head band.

mould should be cleaned regularly with warm soapy water, rinsed thoroughly in clean water, and dried before reconnecting. A piece of wire can be used to remove wax. Condensation in the flexible tubing of postaural aids can be removed by blowing. Many hearing aid centres recommend routine checks of aids every 6 months. Aids should be returned if no longer required.

How to check a hearing aid

If a hearing aid stops working the battery should be checked first of all: when the aid is switched on with the volume turned up a feedback squeal should be heard. Ensure that the ear mould is not blocked and that the flexible tubing of postaural aids or the cord of body worn aids has not perished. Replacements for these can be obtained from hearing aid centres or health centres. If the aid is still not working after these simple tests have been done then it should be returned to the hearing aid centre for repair.

Counselling and rehabilitation

All patients supplied with an aid (including those who have moved into a new area) should be registered with their local hearing aid centre. Many centres operate "open access" and postal systems for repair of aids, and some provide a domiciliary service for elderly or housebound patients.

The provision of an aid is merely one aspect of the rehabilitation of those with impaired hearing. Patients must be taught how to use their aid, and encouraged to contact the hearing aid centre in case of difficulty. In some parts of Britain hearing therapists are available to help patients overcome their initial problems. Children may need special communication and education programmes.[2] Many reasons have been given to explain why hearing aids are underused; these include poor counselling, unrealistic expectations, the degree of hearing loss, background noise, poor speech discrimination, badly fitting ear moulds, and difficulties in handling the aid. Although rehabilitative measures may increase the use of a hearing aid once it has been supplied, this does not necessarily mean that the patient will be more satisfied with it. This raises the question of whether a counselling programme before an aid is supplied would be more effective in improving the hearing aid service.[6]

I thank Mr A Blick, senior chief physiological measurement technician, Audiology Department, St James's University Hospital, Leeds, for his helpful advice in preparing the manuscript.

1 Corcoran AL. A very basic introduction to hearing aids. *Int Rehab Med* 1985;5:67–72.
2 Snashall SE. Deafness in children. *Br J Hosp Med* 1985;33:205–9.
3 Stephens SDG. Hearing aid selection: an integrated approach. *Br J Audiol* 1984;18:199–210.
4 Beswick KBJ. Hearing-impaired patients can always be helped. *Ger Med* 1987;17:55–61.
5 Fountain D. Hearing aids and their care. *Ger Nurs Home Care* 1987;Feb:12–14.
6 Littlejohns P, John AC. Auditory rehabilitation: should we listen to the patient? *Br Med J* 1987;294:1063–4.

Appendix

Useful addresses

The Royal National Institute for the Deaf (RNID), 105 Gower Street, London WC1E 6AH (01 387 8033)

British Association of the Hard of Hearing, 7–11 Armstrong Road, London W3 7JL (01 743 1110)

British Deaf Association, 38 Victoria Place, Carlisle CA1 1HU (0228 48844)

National Deaf Children's Society, 45 Hereford Road, London W2 5AH (01 229 9272)

Useful publications for patients

Available from the Royal National Institute for the Deaf:

RNID Services and Information
Hearing Aids: Questions and Answers
National Health Service Hearing Aids
Visual Doorbell Systems
Aids to Daily Living

Available from the DHSS, PO Box 21, Stanmore, Middlesex HA7 1AY:

General Guidance for Hearing Aid Users
How to Use Your Hearing Aid

Available from British Telecom's Action for Disabled Customers, Room B4036, BT Centre, 81 Newgate Street, London EC1A 7AJ, and from BT shops:

British Telecom's Guide to Equipment and Services for Disabled Customers 1986

Aids for low vision in the elderly

JEFFREY S HILLMAN

Although visual impairment is not caused by increasing age alone, low vision is common in the elderly. The commonest causes of registration of visual handicap are macular degeneration, glaucoma, cataract, and diabetic retinopathy. Many elderly patients with failing vision fear the progression to total loss of sight, and explanation and appropriate reassurance are most important. Emphasise that the eyes do not "wear out" from overuse and the patient can continue to read without harm. Reassure the patient with macular degeneration that, although the detailed central vision used for reading may be lost, the peripheral vision, which is important for mobility, is usually retained and independence need not be lost.

Several aids are available from most major hospital eye departments and from some opticians, but all do require effort and application by the patient if they are to give worthwhile benefit.

Spectacles

It is important that spectacles should be from a recent prescription, and refraction should be checked by an optician about every two years if vision is stable. The power of the reading lenses can be increased to give effective magnification, but as the lenses are strengthened print must be brought closer to the eyes and the positioning of reading matter is critical. The patient must be encouraged to move the print to and fro to find the best distance as print will be out of focus at normal reading distance.

Lighting

The most valuable but least appreciated visual aid is a (60 W) reading light over one shoulder. This usually enables the patient to read at least one size smaller type than with a good ceiling light alone.

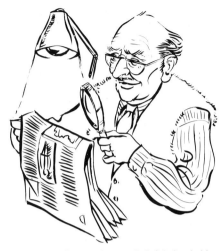

A reading light and hand magnifier are the most helpful visual aids.

Magnifiers

A wide range of magnifiers can be borrowed from hospital eye clinics or bought from opticians, and the patient must be tested to find the most suitable. Stronger magnifiers give increased magnification but at the expense of a closer focus and a reduced field, making it easier for the user to lose the place on the page. The best magnifier is the weakest one which, together with reading spectacles and a good light, enables the patient to read comfortably. The distances between the eyes and the magnifier and the magnifier and the page are critical and the patient must be encouraged to find the best positioning.

For the unsteady hand, a stand magnifier is easy to place at the correct distance from the page, and for the small print in the telephone directory a cylinder bar magnifier helps by elongating the numbers. For tasks requiring the use of both hands, such as knitting, a magnifier held on the chest by a neck cord or held on an adjustable arm can be useful.

Other low vision aids

There are also more sophisticated (and expensive) low vision aids, which are in the form of a high power lens button carried on a spectacle lens or a telescope lens system mounted in one eyepiece of

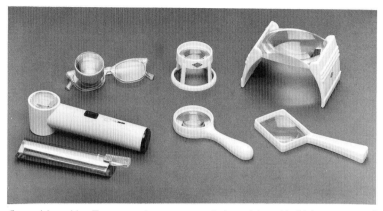

Low vision aids. *Top row:* telescope spectacle low vision aid; high power stand magnifier; low power stand magnifier. *Bottom row:* cylinder bar magnifier and internal illuminated magnifier; high power hand magnifier; medium power hand magnifier.

a spectacle frame. The latter gives magnification with less shortening of the working distance than a simple lens but still needs accurate positioning for real benefit. These aids need specialist testing and are available on free long term loan for hospital eye clinics. Closed circuit television systems are an efficient way of presenting reading matter enlarged without distortion on a television monitor. The high cost may be borne by the Manpower Services Commission if necessary to obtain or maintain a patient in employment.

Large print books

A good selection of books set in large type is available without charge from public libraries, which either hold a stock or will order them for readers.

Talking books

Patients who cannot attain reading vision (N12) may appreciate a talking book, which is available on free loan from social services departments on the recommendation of any doctor; visual handicap registration is not necessary. It is a large tape recorder which accepts special cassettes of a wide range of books. For a small subscription there are also locally organised talking newspaper services co-ordinated by the Talking Newspaper Association, which provide a postal service of an extensive range of newspapers and magazines on standard audio cassettes. Postage is free for those who cannot read.

Visual handicap registration

If vision falls to a level which significantly handicaps the patient it may be appropriate for a consultant ophthalmic surgeon to certify the patient as "partially sighted" or "blind" so that the patient may register with the social services department. *Partial sight registration* implies that the patient is "substantially and permanently handicapped." After registration the patient should be visited by a trained rehabilitation officer who will advise on ways of coping with everyday problems of daily living, mobility, communication, and so on. *Blind registration* implies that the patient is "so blind as to be unable to perform any work for which eyesight is essential." In addition to the advice of a rehabilitation officer, there is increased entitlement to social security benefit and attendance allowance, disabled person's carparking badge (for the patient's carer), free radio, reduced TV licence fee, and the blind person's income tax allowance.

Appendix

Useful addresses

Royal National Institute for the Blind, 224 Great Portland Street, London W1N 6AA (01 388 1266)

North Regional Association for the Blind, Headingley Castle, Headingley Lane, Leeds LS6 2DQ (0532 752666)

South Regional Association for the Blind, 65 Eton Avenue, London NW3 3ET (01 722 9703)

Talking Newspaper Association for the UK, 90 High Street, Heathfield, East Sussex TN21 8JD (04352 6102)

Communication Aids

JAYNE EASTON

Some 800 000 people in the United Kingdom have a severe communication disorder. Many can be helped by communication aids.

Communication aids can be considered as an alternative means of communicating for patients unlikely ever to regain functional speech —for example, those with progressive neurological disorders such as motor neurone disease. They can also be considered as an additional means of communicating—for example, in patients suffering a head injury. Here the communication aid supplements any residual speech in the months before functional speech is achieved. Finally, communication aids can augment any aspect of the speech mechanism that is either weak or absent. For example, amplifiers can increase the volume of a weak voice.

Who can benefit?

Not all patients with a severe speech impairment will benefit from a communication aid. Patients with global dysphasia may not be able to recall the vocabulary required or recognise words, letters, symbols, pictures with which to formulate a message. Patients with non-verbal oral dyspraxia (difficulty in programming the oral musculature) or verbal dyspraxia (difficulty in translating linguistic elements of speech into physical movements) may benefit from the use of an aid, but this will be influenced by their ability to initiate messages and the presence of other concurrent dyspraxic movements (particularly eye movements). Dysarthric patients often gain considerably from a communication aid as theirs is strictly a motor speech disorder, language and vocabulary being intact.

To ensure the provision of the right communication system(s) the speech therapist will carefully assess the patient or may refer him to a communication aids centre (see appendix). There staff will determine the optimum system(s) and train the patient to use the equipment effectively. Many of these centres exhibit a large display of communication aids.

Communication systems available

Low tech systems

"Low tech" systems include picture and symbol charts for those who have difficulty in understanding or expressing themselves through the written word. Some use simple black and white line drawings; others use photographs. A number of alphabet cards and word charts with a preselected vocabulary are commercially available, but others are often tailored by the therapist to include vocabulary applicable to the individual. Sign languages are another form of "low tech" communication. The system chosen will depend on the patient's physical ability to control hand movements, his or her memory for shapes, and the support of others, who will also need to learn the system.

High tech systems

Direct selection — There are small portable communication aids that incorporate mini keyboards — for example, the Canon Communicator or the Memowriter. The Lightwriter and Helpmate use a normal sized keyboard but have special keys for those with limited physical abilities. Large keyboards are also available for those with poor fine motor control who require a large target area. Some direct selection communication aids can be operated by a headpointer, mouthstick, or light beam. Sometimes words or symbols are used to compose the message, rather than letters; this tends to speed up the rate of communication but limits the user's vocabulary. The message can appear on a visual display or be printed out or spoken by an electronic voice.

Scanning — Very physically handicapped patients who cannot point may need a switch operated scanning method. Any reliable motor action may be harnessed to operate a switch which can be used to start and stop a light or mechanical pointer scanning over a number of vocabulary items and thus indicating a message. This may enable a very disabled person to use a word processor without ever having to touch the keyboard. Switches allow access to computer software such as adapted word processing packages and games, as well as keyboard emulators (which transfer keyboard functions on to a visual display unit where they are scanned by a cursor). There are also portable scanning mechanisms which can be used more specifically as an

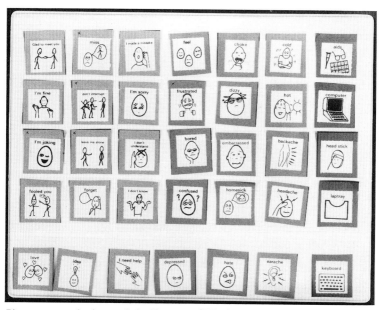

Picture communication symbols. (Courtesy of Winslow Press.)

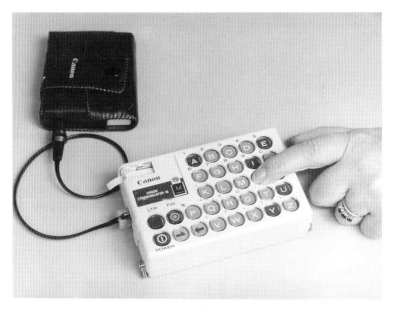

Canon Communicator. (Courtesy of Canon (UK) Ltd.)

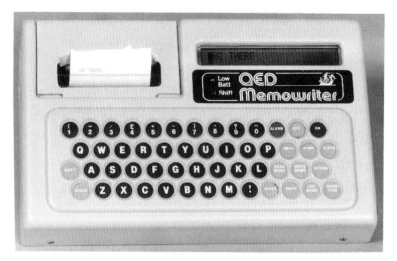

Memowriter. (Courtesy of QED (Quest Educational Designs) Ltd.)

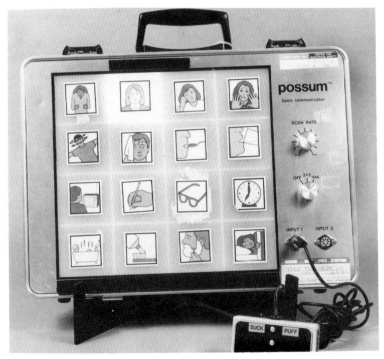

Possum 4/16 scanning communicator with pictures. (Courtesy of Possum Controls Ltd.)

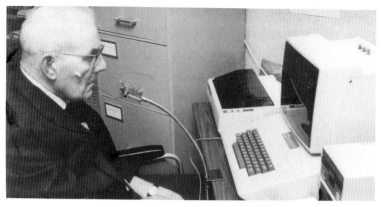

Minimal head movement permits operation of sensitive cheek switches, which enable patient to use an adapted word processor.

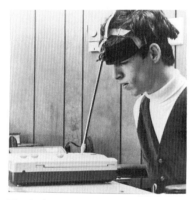

Headpointer.

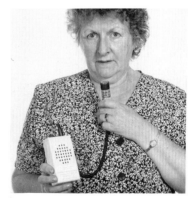

Mediquip speech amplifier. (Courtesy of Mediquip Surgical Supplies Ltd.)

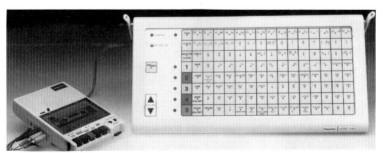

Phonic mirror handivoice speech synthesiser. (Courtesy of P C Werth Ltd.)

alternative to speech, such as the Light Talker and Toucan; again these provide multiple outputs—printed, visual, or spoken.

Telephone aids—A speech amplifier may be all that is required, but if modifications are needed to cater for a person's poor motor control or if the patient's voice is too weak British Telecom produces a booklet, *Aids for the Disabled*, which may help. Speech synthesisers can be used for telephone conversations. The quality varies enormously, some having a human sounding voice but only a limited vocabulary. The Claudius Converse marketed by British Telecom, for example, has 64 prestored phrases that can be spoken in a male or female voice. Other synthesisers enable the patient to use an infinite vocabulary but sound robotic. Equipment is also available that allows patients to type their message into a special typewriter that relays its contents on to a visual display incorporated into similar equipment at the receiver's end.

How to encourage the use of the equipment

- Make sure the equipment is accessible to the patient. Remember that he or she may not be able to ask for it.
- Encourage the use of communication systems by conversing with the patient, not admiring the equipment and directing your conversation to the accompanying relative or spouse.
- Allow time for patients to communicate; do not frustrate them by answering your own questions, guessing ahead, and closing the conversation before they have had a chance to complete the message in answer to your first question. If you have not time to wait ask patients to prepare any questions they may have for you in advance.
- Adopt a positive attitude towards the use of communication equipment. Comments relating to "Dalek-like voices," "toys," and "gadgets" may discourage acceptance. Remember it takes a lot of courage to use this equipment outside a cossetted clinical environment.
- Encourage patients to use any speech they may have in addition to the communication aid.

Useful references

Communication aids: a guide for people who have difficulty in speaking. London: Research Institute for Consumer Affairs, 1984.
Wilshire ER, comp. *Equipment for disabled people: communication.* Oxford: Oxfordshire Health Authority, 1987.

Appendix

Communication aids centres

These centres, funded jointly by the DHSS and the Royal Association for Disability and Rehabilitation (RADAR), are at the following addresses:

Frenchay Hospital, Bristol BS16 1LE (0272 565656: ext 2151)
Charing Cross Hospital, London W6 8RF (01 748 2040: ext 3064)
The Wolfson Centre, London WC1N 2AP (01 837 7618: ext 9)
The Dene Centre, Castle Farm Road, Newcastle upon Tyne (091 284 0480)
Boulton Road, West Bromwich B70 6NN (021 553 0908)
Rookwood Hospital, Cardiff CF5 2YN (0222 566281)

Other centres

Communication Aids Centre, St George's Hospital, Sheffield 10
William Merritt Disabled Living Centre, St Mary's Hospital, Leeds LS12 3QE (0532 793140)
Leicester Communication Aids Centre, Yeoman House, Yeoman Street, Leicester (0533 56811)
Truro Communication Aids Centre, Treliske Hospital, Truro (0872 74242: ext 520)
Southampton Communications Aids Centre, Southampton General Hospital, Southampton SO9 4XY (0703 777222)
Scottish Centre for Technology for the Communication Impaired, Victoria Infirmary, Glasgow G42 9TY (041 649 4545)
Communication Advice Centre, Musgrave Park Hospital, Belfast BT9 7JB (0232 669501: ext 561/555)

Education

Special Education Microelectronics Resource Centres (SEMERCS) specialise in software for children with special educational needs and train teachers in its application. Centres are found at the following colleges:

Bristol Polytechnic, Bristol BS6 6UZ (0272 741251)
Manchester College of Higher Education, Manchester M13 0JA (0612 259054)
Newcastle Polytechnic, Newcastle upon Tyne NE7 7XA (0632 665057)
Dane Centre, Melbourne Road, Ilford, Essex IG1 4HT

The ACE Centre (Aids for Communication in Education) is also concerned with the use of microelectronic communication aids in education and provides an assessment and information service:

Ormerod School, Waynflete Road, Oxford OX3 8DD (0865 61501)

The National ACCESS Centre provides detailed assessments of students in relation to further education, training, and employment:

Hereward College of Further Education, Coventry CV4 9SW (0203 461231)

Provision of equipment

The National Health Service can supply communication aids on a district's "aids and appliances" budget. This requires a consultant's signature and depends on availability of funds within the district.

19

The Department of Health and Social Security will supply a limited number of aids to patients from central funding. To qualify for this equipment patients must also be very severely physically handicapped.

Social services departments must, under the Chronically Sick and Disabled Persons Act 1970 section 2, assess the need for equipment required by individuals in the community. If they accept that there is a need in an individual case social services departments do not have to meet the need in the way it is requested and they can charge.

Local education authorities have a statutory responsibility to educate children and may therefore acquire communication equipment for a child if it is thought to be essential for his or her education. Communication systems remain the property of the local education authority, who are not always sufficiently flexible to allow the child to use the equipment at home or when he or she leaves school permanently.

The Manpower Services Commission will provide special aids to enable a disabled person to obtain or retain suitable employment. The equipment provided is only for use at work.

Loan facilities—The communication aids centres and some speech therapy departments hold banks of equipment available for long term loan by those who are progressively ill and whose needs are constantly changing. After assessment short term loans can be arranged to establish the suitability of any equipment recommended, before funds are sought for its permanent procurement. Equipment can be borrowed from various agencies, such as the charity Special Equipment and Aids for Living (SEQUAL). Some disorder related charities—for example, the Motor Neurone Disease Association—also have banks of equipment from which they can loan communication aids.

Charity funding—With limited local and national government spending the speech handicapped person's needs may not be met by statutory provision and voluntary organisations may have to be approached, such as the Spastics Society.

Private purchase—Equipment bought privately for use by a disabled person is zero rated for value added tax on the presentation of a suitable declaration (Customs and Excise VAT Leaflets 701/6/81 and 701/7/81 (HMSO)); a supporting letter from a doctor is no longer needed.

Voluntary organisations—The Rehabilitation Engineering Movement Advisory Panel (REMAP) is a voluntary organisation whose aim is to design, make, or adapt aids for handicapped people, many being custom built to suit the individual's needs.

ACTIVE is another voluntary group that makes and adapts equipment for play, teaching, recreation, and communication.

Collars and Corsets

G J HUSTON

Collars

Soft collars may be prescribed for the management of neck pain resulting from cervical spondylosis or to provide comfort and limit neck movement after road accidents. They have not been shown to be better than placebo treatments[1] and restrict neck movement only minimally.[2]

Convention suggests that if pain is severe a firm collar should be worn during the day and a soft one at night. There are no studies to support the use of firm or rigid collars if the cervical spine is stable; and the minimum effective period of daily wear is unknown, as is patient compliance. Potential disadvantages such as discomfort, excess heat, habituation, or predisposition of the frail elderly to falls remain unstudied.

Rigid collars do not restrict intervertebral movement smoothly and may produce localised areas of flattening or reversed lordosis. The use of such collars by patients with an unstable rheumatoid spine therefore requires specialist assessment of the risks and benefits, and precise fitting.

Patients will expect to wash the covering of a collar. If the covering is removable and dries easily one collar will suffice because 75% of patients with stable cervical spines have been cured or are improving four weeks after the start of treatment.[1] The collar will therefore probably be required for a maximum of two months. Some patients find that wearing a silk scarf over the collar adds to comfort. A collar that causes increased pain should be altered or abandoned. Soft collars are usually prescribed at consultant clinics. There is no prescription charge to the patient, but the charge to the National Health Service is about £10 to £12. A serviceable collar can be made in the general practitioner's surgery using a pair of scissors and materials prescribable on FP10 forms.[3] Other possible sources of collars are casualty departments or open access physiotherapy departments.

Lumbar supports

Lumbar supports with rigid inserts are used in the treatment of back pain and sciatica. A small trial of 19 patients suggested that any beneficial effect was due to the limitation of lumbar movement produced by rigid inserts in the back of the support.[4] If a corset extends beyond the thoracolumbar junction it may, paradoxically, fail to immobilise the lumbar spine.[5] The use of corsets to alleviate back pain and sciatica in patients with stable lumbar spines is not supported by multicentre trials.[6 7] Pain deriving from a spondylolisthesis may, however, respond more favourably than back pain with no specific identifiable cause.[8]

Concern has been expressed over the possibility of disuse atrophy of the lumbar muscles with the use of lumbar supports, and some authors deprecate their use,[9] though no objective evidence of their harmful effects has been produced. Corsets are best avoided in young people, particularly if there is even a remote possibility of ankylosing spondylitis. There are no studies of patient compliance with the use of lumbar supports or of the minimum effective period of daily wear.

Corsets are usually available only from hospitals, under the direction of a consultant. They are fitted by an orthotist, who usually makes subsequent adjustments and modifications to ensure the comfort of the patient. They are normally worn throughout the day. It is permissible for the patient to wear a light cotton vest under the corset. There is a prescription charge of £15, which is waived for inpatients or those in the usual exemption groups. The cost of a made to measure corset is between £50 and £60, but ready made corsets start at about £20.

Conclusion

Current information suggests that soft collars and lumbar supports act primarily as placebos in patients with stable spines. But they may be a less expensive means of providing a physical placebo than physiotherapy—though this is yet another unstudied area. Probably they have a useful minor role in the management of patients with neck and back pain who do not wish to take simple analgesics.

1 British Association of Physical Medicine. Pain in the neck and arm: a multicentre trial of the effects of physiotherapy. *Br Med J* 1966;i:253–8.
2 Colachis SC, Strohm BR, Ganter EL. Cervical spine motion in normal women: radiographic study of the effect of cervical collars. *Arch Phys Med Rehabil* 1973;54:161–9.

3 Jacobs SM, Griffiths DC. *Treatment room nursing—a handbook for nursing sisters working in general practice, schools and industry.* London: Blackwell, 1976.

4 Million R, Haavik Nilsen K, Jayson MIV, Baker RD. Evaluation of low back pain and assessment of lumbar corsets with and without back supports. *Ann Rheum Dis* 1981;**40**:449–54.

5 Norton PL, Brown T. The immobilizing efficiency of back braces. *J Bone Joint Surg* 1957;**39A**:111–38.

6 Doran DML, Newell DJ. Manipulation in treatment of low back pain: a multicentre study. *Br Med J* 1975;ii:161–4.

7 Coxhead CE, Inskip H, Mead TW, *et al.* Multicentre trial of physiotherapy in the management of sciatic symptoms. *Lancet* 1981;i:1065–8.

8 Willner S. Effect of a rigid brace on back pain. *Acta Orthop Scand* 1985;**56**:40–2.

9 Quinet RJ, Hadler NM. Diagnosis and treatment of backache. *Semin Arthritis Rheum* 1979;**8**:261–87.

Elastic Stockings

ALAN J WHITLEY

If the valves of deep veins or perforated veins in the leg become incompetent or deep veins are occluded by thrombosis high venous pressure develops during standing and walking. The dermal capillaries subsequently become distended and the high pressures may force macromolecules (including fibrinogen) into the extravascular space. This causes tightly stretched, pigmented hard skin in the gaiter area of the leg (lipodermatosclerosis), a forerunner of gravitational ulceration.[1] Elastic support stockings overcome the effects of prolonged venous hypertension.

Elastic compression decreases the superficial venous pressure, increases the upward flow in the unoccluded deep and superficial veins, and raises local interstitial pressure. Compression of the leg also relieves discomfort by preventing excessive venous distension caused by extensive superficial varices.[2]

Elastic stockings are the commonest corrective treatment for deep venous insufficiency, yet some patients refuse to wear them because the stockings may not relieve discomfort, may fail to resolve oedema, and may even make their symptoms worse. These failures usually occur because the stockings do not fit well. Elastic stockings should provide a graduated compression, exerting most pressure at the ankle, less pressure at the calf, and least pressure in the thigh. The greater the compression gradient between the ankle and calf the lower the ambulatory venous pressure in the deep veins.[3]

Choice of stocking

Since this chapter was published as an article in the *British Medical Journal*, on 6 February 1988, the specifications for hosiery have been changed for the first time in 20 years. Revised standards were introduced by the Department of Health and Social Security on 1 April 1988. Under the new system "compression hosiery" (formerly "elastic stockings") must conform to BSS 6612. This is an important advance since specific compressions at the ankle can now be guaranteed; these are given in the table.

Class	Pressure at ankle (mm Hg)
I	14–17
II	18–24
III	25–35

Conformity with BSS 6612 can be checked with a HATRA hose pressure tester. But the pressures are determined by the relative sizes of the ankle and calf—and, where applicable, the thigh. They can thus be guaranteed in the standard range of stock sizes for a wide spectrum of leg shapes.

Class I compression hosiery is suitable for patients with early varices, early venous dysfunction, post-phlebitic syndrome, deep vein thrombosis, for those who have had superficial vein transplants during coronary bypass surgery, or for the prevention of varicose veins in pregnancy.

Class II is suitable for patients with moderate varices, oedema, or post-phlebitic syndrome.

Class III is suitable for patients with severe varices, severe oedema, or deep venous dysfunction.

The hosiery is supplied in below knee or thigh length. It is better to prescribe thigh length hosiery for a woman who is used to wearing suspenders; but for women who wear trousers or for men below knee stockings are acceptable. Open toed stockings are available as well as fully footed ones. The open toed kind should, of course, be prescribed for patients whose feet are grossly deformed.

Practical problems

Preservation of the elasticity of the stockings depends on how they are washed and dried. Washing instructions are quite specific: the water must be lukewarm; the stockings must not be wrung or twisted; they should be dried naturally, away from artifical heat or sunlight. This means that two sets of stockings must be provided for each patient. Stockings should be replaced regularly: Scholl recommends replacement every three months.

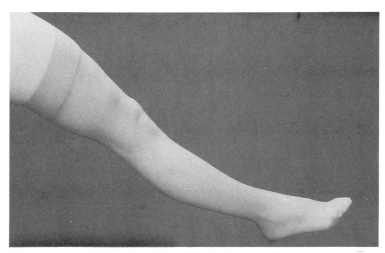

To ensure correct fitting, the ankle, calf, and thigh circumference, as appropriate, should be measured accurately and as early in the day as practical to eliminate the effects of oedema caused by upright posture. (Courtesy of Scholl Consumer Products Ltd.)

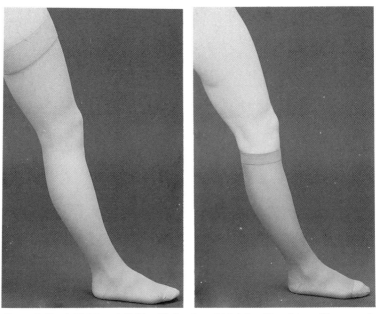

Correctly fitted thigh length (*left*) and below knee (*right*) class II stockings. (Courtesy of Scholl Consumer Products Ltd.)

If the patient is elderly and has restricted flexion of the hip joints it may be impossible for her to reach down to her feet to put on the stockings. Stocking aids (provided by occupational therapists) cannot usually cope with the strength of a standard weight elastic stocking. Therefore arthritic patients may have difficulty in putting on strong elastic stockings. Many patients who have suffered strokes also cannot put them on.

A problem for the many elderly women who do not wear suspender belts or corsets is that the thigh part of their stockings comes down and hangs loosely around their knees. For them, class I elastic below knee stockings should be considered.

Elastic stockings should be taken off at night before the patient gets into bed, and they should be put on in the morning before she starts to walk. Ideally, they should be kept by the side of the bed and the patient should put them on while she is still lying down.

The stockings should be turned inside out, except for the foot up to the heel. The foot should then be inserted into the stocking until the heel of the stocking corresponds with the heel of the foot. The stocking should then be worked up over the ankle, pulling it up in folds a little at a time. It should be removed by peeling off, not by rolling or pulling at the ankle (Scholl *Hosiery and Dressing* booklet). The fingernails should be free from rough edges, which might cause damage to the stocking or, more seriously, to the fragile skin of the leg.

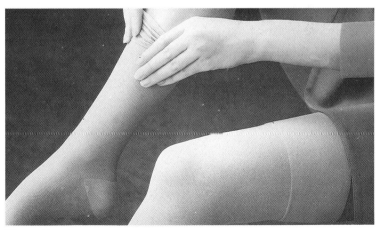

The stocking should be worked up over the ankle, pulling it in folds a little at a time. (Courtesy of Scholl Consumer Products Ltd.)

Prescription guidelines

(1) Explain to patients why elastic stockings would be helpful.

(2) If they agree to try them suggest that they should take the prescription to the pharmacist and that they should ask him for a measurement form. Patients can measure their ankles and calves at home. However, surgical appliance suppliers usually have staff on their premises who will take measurements.

(3) If you think a patient can manage standard weight stockings and is used to wearing suspenders prescribe *standard weight, thigh length*, class II.

(4) If not prescribe *thigh length*, class I.

(5) For women who do not wear suspenders or for men, prescribe *below knee*, class II.

(6) Prescribe one pair and ask the patient to return after two weeks for reappraisal.

(7) If the stockings are satisfactory prescribe a second pair, explaining the need to wear them permanently and to have them replaced every three months, or when the elasticity deteriorates.

1 Burnand KG, Clemenson G, Morland M, Jarrett PGM, Browse NL. Venous lipodermatosis: treatment by fibrinolytic enhancement and elastic compression. *Br Med J* 1980;**280**:7–11.
2 Burnand KG, Layer GT. Graduated elastic stockings. *Br Med J* 1986;**293**:224–5.
3 Horner J, Fernandes E, Fernandes J, Nicolaides AN. Value of graduated compression stockings in deep venous insufficiency. *Br Med J* 1980;**280**:820–1.

Appendix

Current cost of elastic stockings

Class I:	thigh stockings	£5·30 per pair
	below knee stockings	£5·00 per pair
Class II:	thigh stockings, normal size	£8·20 per pair
	below knee stockings	£7·30 per pair
Class III:	thigh stockings, normal size	£9·70 per pair

Special Footwear

E G WHITE

Special footwear (also called "orthopaedic" or "surgical" footwear) may be supplied free of charge to patients in whom deformity of the feet or legs makes ordinary shoes unsuitable. If possible the patient's own shoes are adapted, but when this cannot be done ready made or made to measure special footwear may be provided. Various orthoses (calipers, splints, and appliances) may be incorporated into the footwear or space made available for them. Special footwear cannot be provided for an allergic condition or when left and right feet are of different sizes, unless other special features are needed.

Indications

The main function of special footwear is to accommodate deformed feet, providing a protective covering and a sound base for walking. It may also help to relieve pain or to compensate for inequality in leg length.

In older patients common problems are bunions, hammer toes, and rheumatoid arthritis. Extra space for the toes is needed in these conditions. Children with neuromuscular disorders such as cerebral palsy and spina bifida commonly require special shoes. When sensation is impaired openings in the shoes extending to the toes help to prevent the toes from curling under when footwear is put on. Juvenile chronic arthritis affecting the foot may also necessitate special footwear.

A number of modifications can be made to relieve pain or improve function: insoles may be added to redistribute weight and relieve pressure; insoles with extra padding placed behind the metatarsal heads are used in metatarsalgia; valgus supports are built up under the medial arch for conditions like valgus heels—though their use as a prop in children with pes planovalgus ("flat foot") is best avoided.

When prescribing insoles it is important to allow enough depth in the shoe to accommodate them.

The heel and sole of the shoe may also be modified. A wedge of soling material added to the edge of the heel or sole and tapering towards the middle may help in cases where the heel goes into valgus or varus on weight bearing; the wedge is positioned medially for valgus and laterally for varus. For patients with valgus ankles the heel may also be extended along the inner border of the shoe to support the instep or extended outwards (floated) on the medial side. A plastic heel cup worn inside a child's shoe can hold the heel straight. In patients with pes planovalgus such modifications may help when shoe wear is excessive, but whether they make any long term difference to the condition is contentious. A lateral heel float may be useful for people with recurrent inversion sprains.

In patients with hallux rigidus pain can be relieved by adding a rocker sole, a built up sole tapering to the toe; it allows the foot to rock forwards, thus eliminating extension of the first toe.

Sockets for calipers can be added if calipers are needed to improve ankle stability or control foot drop. A raise may be added if one leg is shorter than the other. Complete compensation is not usually attempted; a difference of one centimetre is acceptable. The heel should be raised more than the sole, which should taper towards the toe. Velcro may be used to help patients who have difficulty with fastenings.

How to obtain special footwear

Special footwear is not available on prescription from general practitioners: it can only be obtained through hospital based services.

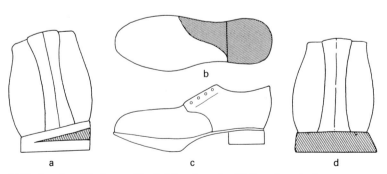

(a) Heel wedge; (b) elongated heel; (c) rocker sole; (d) floated out heel.

Patients not already receiving hospital treatment should initially be referred by their general practitioner to a hospital consultant, usually an orthopaedic surgeon or rheumatologist. Guidelines for the prescription of footwear are given in a handbook[1] available to hospital appliance departments. The hospital appliance officer is the next link in the chain. In most hospitals his duties are primarily administrative and the manufacture of the footwear is contracted out to a private supplier. The appliance officer arranges for an orthotist (who is trained in the measurement and fitting of all types of orthoses) from

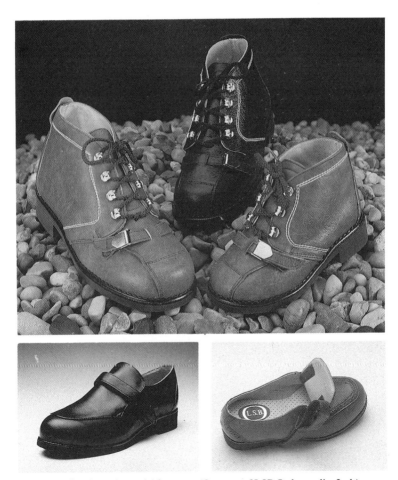

Examples of ready made special footwear. (Courtesy of LSB Orthopaedics Ltd.)

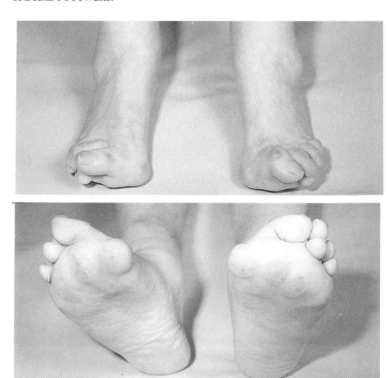

Patient with deformed rheumatoid feet. (Courtesy of LSB Orthopaedics Ltd.)

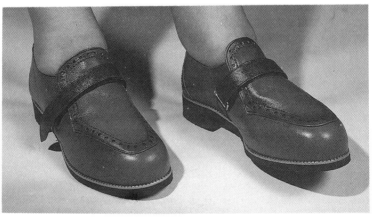

Ready made deep rounded stock shoe with velcro fastener. (Courtesy of LSB Orthopaedics Ltd.)

the private contractor to see the patient and take measurements. If deformities are gross a plaster cast may be made. The footwear is made in the appliances workshop to the specification given in a detailed form filled in by the orthotist. Insoles and straightforward shoe modifications should be available in two weeks or so and made to measure shoes within two months. Priority is given to all orders for children's footwear and first orders for adults' footwear. Delays in fulfilling orders should be brought to the attention of the appliance officer: if necessary he will consider an alternative supplier.

Made to measure footwear

Made to measure footwear is available in a number of styles and colours. Possible additions include raises, insoles, and sockets for calipers. If extra support is needed at the ankle boots may be supplied. After an initial session at which measurements are taken the patient is usually required to visit again for a fitting before the footwear is finished. When it is supplied he is asked to try it out for several weeks to make certain that it fits satisfactorily. If it does, a second pair of shoes is made up to the same order. Usually two pairs are provided, but further ones can be ordered if needed. Repairs to special footwear are free of charge, and requests for these can be made by the patient directly to the appliance department. If the patient's condition is stable replacement pairs can be provided for up to five years without the patient's seeing the consultant again. There is no limit to the number of replacement pairs a patient can have, the criterion for replacement being the serviceability of the footwear. Children and active adults may need frequent replacements and should always have two usable pairs available.

Ready made special footwear

Ready made special footwear comes in stock sizes. It has extra width or depth to accommodate deformities. This is useful for forefoot deformities such as hallux valgus and hammer toes. There is a range of makes and styles and most are suitable for orthopaedic alterations. Depth may be adjusted by the use of extra insoles. For children a range of special boots is available with such features as lacing to the toes. Ready made special footwear can be provided much more quickly than footwear that is made to measure and at considerably lower cost. Even without additions, made to measure shoes cost the National Health Service about £180, whereas ready made shoes cost from £50 to £60.

Shoe adaptations

When it is possible to adapt standard footwear patients will be asked to provide shoes at their own expense, but the adaptations will be carried out free of charge. However, not all shoes bought in the high street can be adapted; the patient should therefore seek the advice of the orthotist before buying. Repairs not affecting the adaptations must be paid for by the patient.

Patient satisfaction

A survey of special footwear showed a high level of patient satisfaction, with 82% satisfied or highly satisfied overall.[2] None the less, some problems did occur. Discomfort was experienced at some time by 30%, and 29% had difficulty putting the footwear on. Nineteen per cent were dissatisfied with the style or colour. Supply arrangements were complained of by 13%, especially the long delay between being measured and receiving the finished footwear (34% waited over two months). Thirty five per cent considered that they did not have enough pairs of shoes.

The range of footwear available has slowly improved in recent years and patients should be given as much choice as the constraints of their underlying foot problems allow. An understanding of what is required and close cooperation between the prescriber and orthotist should ensure that the patient gets maximum benefit from the most appropriate footwear.

1 Department of Health and Social Security. *Provision of medical and surgical appliances.* London: HMSO, 1983. (Booklet MHM 50.)
2 Bainbridge S. *National Health surgical footwear—a study of patient satisfaction.* London: HMSO, 1979.

Further reading

Helfet AJ, Gruebel Lee DM, eds. *Disorders of the foot.* Philadelphia: Lippincott, 1980.
Rose GK. *Orthotics, principles and practice.* London: Heinemann Medical Books, 1986.
Stewart J, Hallett J. *Traction and orthopaedic appliances.* Edinburgh: Churchill Livingstone, 1983.
Hughes J, ed. *Footwear and footcare for disabled children.* London: Disabled Living Foundation, 1982.
Hughes J. *Footwear and footcare for adults.* London: Disabled Living Foundation, 1983.

Walking sticks

GRAHAM P MULLEY

The doctor's stick with its gold handle was once a symbol of his profession, and at the turn of the century a nobleman was not considered fully dressed without his jaunty stick. Nowadays, sticks have little social meaning. Indeed, elderly ladies may feel too proud to be seen using them. Yet the walking stick can be as important a tool to a person with joint disease or problems with balance as golf clubs, skis, and rackets are to the sportsman.

Indications for walking sticks

Some elderly people use sticks to proclaim their frailty. Unfortunately, some need to carry them as a defensive weapon. White sticks help identify those who are blind. Walking sticks reduce the fear of instability and can aid locomotion in hemiplegia. They relieve pain by giving support and therefore improve mobility. In degenerative joint conditions affecting the legs and after hip operations the stick aids walking by transmitting some of the body's weight through the arm. A typical patient with osteoarthritis of the hip will take 13·5 kg of his weight through his stick and this greatly diminishes the static forces on the affected joint.

Before prescribing a stick it must be established that the patient has enough strength and control in the upper arm and that the arm and hand are free from any joint condition which would be exacerbated by using the stick. In unilateral disease one stick should suffice, but two sticks (which give better balance and weight relief[1]) may be needed in bilateral disease.

How to choose the correct stick

We should give as much care to assessing a stick as we would to fitting shoes[2] and should pay particular attention to the material, length, handle, and tip.

Material

A descendant of the shepherd's crook, the wooden stick has a traditional quality denied to utilitarian metal sticks. Wood is cheaper and usually lighter. Many sticks are bought privately (from country fairs or, curiously, tobacconists); others are inherited. Some are obtained from hospitals or social service departments. Wooden sticks have a curved handle which allows the stick to be placed on the forearm or coat hook. The wood should be examined for splintering or decay. The shaft should not be too flexible or it will feel insecure and may not withstand the increased load engendered by using stairs.

Lightweight aluminium sticks are more robust and their length is adjustable. They do not fracture and are fitted with plastic or rubber handles contoured to the individual.[3]

Length

As a general rule the correct length of a stick from the top of the handle to the tip is equal to the distance from the proximal wrist crease to the ground.[4] The user should be standing erect, wearing everyday shoes, and the elbow should be flexed to 15° when the stick is held at rest. This allows full extension of the arm when the stick is placed ahead during walking. If a considerable weight is to be transmitted through the stick a slightly longer stick may be helpful: studies on sticks fitted with strain gauges have shown that the angle at which most weight is transmitted through the arm is at 30° of elbow flexion. A stick of optimum length prevents the user leaning towards the stick (which occurs if the stick is too short) or away from it (if it is too long). It also ensures that the stick can be placed in front of the user without his bending forwards during walking.

In a survey of sticks used by elderly people it was found that two thirds of the sticks were too long.[4] An excessively long stick does not allow adequate weight transmission through the arm. It also raises the shoulder, producing an unsightly appearance, and increases elbow flexion, with greater demands on the triceps. The undue force on the wrist may cause median nerve compression.[1] If a stick is too long do not immediately reduce its length or replace it: someone who has become used to a long stick may feel insecure if it is suddenly shortened. Here an adjustable metal stick, shortened little by little, may be useful. Sometimes physiotherapists intentionally give long sticks to hemiplegic patients, who tend to take much of their weight through the contralateral leg. By using a long stick in the unaffected arm, the patient is encouraged to bear more weight through the

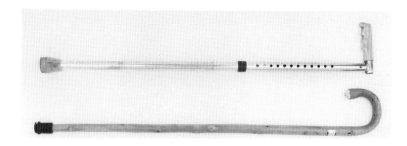

Top: Aluminium stick with grips on the straight plastic handle. Note the adjustable length. *Bottom:* Wooden stick with curved handle.

affected side, thus producing a better gait pattern. Therefore it is wise to consult the therapist before altering a stroke victim's stick.

The handle

For comfort, the handle should be of the correct shape and diameter. The curved handles of wooden sticks are adequate for the person using a stick for a short time. They also have practical advantages: they can be used to retrieve dropped items, turn switches on and off, and pull up underclothing. However, curved handles concentrate pressure on a small area at the base of the palm and they are not recommended for those with chronic arthritis.[2]

Some aluminium sticks have a straight handle of greater diameter with grips on the plastic handle. Other shapes are available: a handle with a swan neck may be better for those with balance problems, as the centre of balance is brought directly over the stick. Specially moulded plastic Fischer handles are helpful for patients with rheumatism.

If the diameter of the stick is too small the close contact between fingers and palm will cause discomfort. Foam, felt, and other materials may be used to expand the handle, making gripping easier for the arthritic patient. In practice these simple modifications are rarely considered.[4]

The tip

Metal tips were first introduced to prevent the wood at the end of the stick from splitting. They were called ferrules (a word derived from the old French word *virelle*, a bracelet). Sticks with plain wooden ends or metal tips tend to slip. All walking sticks should

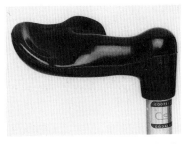 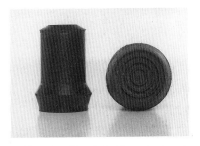

Moulded plastic Fischer handle for patients with rheumatoid hands.

Rubber tips (ferrules). Note the broad base *(side view)* and the concentric rings on the base which give a good grip.

therefore be fitted with a soft rubber tip which will reduce slipping and perhaps reduce the risk of falls. Several designs are available, most having flared sides and a flat base. Rounded rubber tips are to be avoided. Tips with concentric rings or cylindrical studs on the base are preferred. Rubber tips become worn with regular use and Nichols and Mowat[1] argued that it was as important to change worn ferrules on a stick as to replace worn tyres on a car.

Regrettably, rubber tips tend to slip on wet pavements, snow, and ice. The rubber tip has been the single most important development in walking stick safety. A tip which was safer in winter conditions would be another important advance. At present the patient has to maintain stability as best he can in adverse conditions by walking more slowly and holding the stick as near vertical as possible.

Holding a stick: which hand?

Many people wrongly hold the stick in the ipsilateral hand.[5] In normal walking, the leg and opposite arm move together. This reciprocal pattern is abolished if the stick is held in the wrong hand and an unnatural amphibious walking pattern will be produced, the centre of gravity moving markedly from side to side with each step.[6] The stick should therefore be held in the contralateral hand. Here it provides a wider base, which gives better stability and allows a more normal gait.[7] However, some people will always want to use their dominant hand and attempts to alter this tendency will be unsuccessful. In hemiplegic patients, too, the stick should be held in the contralateral hand, where it increases confidence and encourages a better pattern of walking.

It is unusual to see a parkinsonian patient with a stick. In this condition the use of two sticks can be helpful: a stick held in each hand facilitates truncal rotation and encourages the normal reciprocal walking pattern.

Tripods and tetrapods

Although most sticks have a single stem, pyramid sticks (with three or four legs) are more stable[1 6] and may be used by older people with poor balance. The tetrapod is said to be more stable than a tripod. These sticks are less helpful on uneven terrain or in rooms where there is little space for manoeuvre. The wide base may not fit stairs. They produce a halting, almost crablike gait.

I am grateful to my physiotherapist colleagues, Rosemary Taylor and Julie Isaac, for their helpful advice.

1 Nichols PJR, Mowat AG. *Splints, walking aids and appliances for the arthritic patient.* London: Arthritis and Rheumatism Council, 1972. (Reports on Rheumatic Diseases No 48.)
2 Chalmers J. Walking sticks used by the elderly. *Br Med J* 1982;**285**:57–8.
3 Michaelson P. Walking sticks used by the elderly. *Br Med J* 1982;**285**:58.
4 Sainsbury R, Mulley GP. Walking sticks used by the elderly. *Br Med J* 1982;**284**:1751.
5 Leary PR. Walking sticks used by the elderly. *Br Med J* 1982;**285**:85.
6 Jebsen RH. Use and abuse of ambulation aids. *JAMA* 1967;**199**:63–8.
7 Cress RH. Ambulation aids for the elderly. *Med Instr* 1982;**16**:169–72.

Recommended reading

Wilshire ER, comp. *Equipment for the disabled: walking aids.* Oxford: Oxfordshire Health Authority, 1987.

Wheelchairs

JOHN B YOUNG

There are about 400 000 wheelchair users in the United Kingdom, more than half of whom are over 65. The bewildering range of available wheelchairs may make selection seem difficult. However, most patients can be helped by either a standard self propelling wheelchair or an attendant (push) wheelchair. Patients with abnormal postures, complex disabilities, or demanding mobility requirements are best referred for specialist assessment.[1]

Sources

Wheelchairs can be obtained on indefinite free loan from the Department of Health and Social Security through disablement service centres. Alternatively, wheelchairs may be privately purchased from the manufacturer or from a local retailer. Short term wheelchair provision—for example, for holidays—can be arranged from the health authority's medical loans department, or from the Red Cross.

Ordering

DHSS wheelchairs are obtained by posting a completed appliance order form 5 (AOF5G) to the nearest disablement service centre. The form indicates the wheelchair thought most appropriate and requires a doctor's signature. An unsuitable wheelchair is a source of great frustration; therefore advice should be sought if there is uncertainty about completing the form. Advice can be obtained by referring the patient directly to the centre and requesting an assessment. The patient will then be asked to attend a wheelchair clinic or will be seen at home. Advice is also available from community occupational therapists employed by the local authority; they will assess the patient at home. Most districts will also have an interested specialist available—for example, a rheumatologist or geriatrician—who can refer patients and will usually assess them in consultation with a hospital physiotherapist and occupational therapist.

Prescribing

Defining the mobility need

A wheelchair is a practical solution to practical problems. These need to be identified and discussed with the patient for a wheelchair to be successful. What does the patient wish to do that he cannot do now? The answer will indicate whether the wheelchair is for use indoors or outdoors, or both; whether it is for occasional or constant use; whether it should be self propelling or of the push type; whether it should be manual or electric; and the accessories that are likely to be needed.

Selecting a wheelchair

Over 66 models are available from the DHSS and are described in the *Handbook of Wheelchairs (MHM 408)*.[2] The non-specialist should become familiar with the following general purpose chairs that meet the mobility needs of most adult patients.

Model 9L is a transit or pushchair which has small rear wheels and is pushed by an attendant (the L stands for "lightweight").

Model 8L is self propelling: the user moves the chair with the large rear wheels. However, it can also be pushed by an attendant.

Model 8BL is a slightly smaller version of model 8L. It is useful in confined spaces.

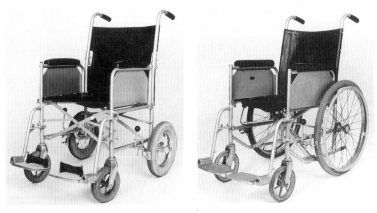

Wheelchairs: model 9L *(left)* and model 8L *(right)*.

These three wheelchairs are for indoor or outdoor use. They fold for compact storage, have pneumatic tyres (for comfort), lever brakes, and detachable footrest plates. They fit into most car boots, but many people find them heavy and awkward to lift (weight approximately 16 kg). Model 8 chairs have armrests which can be removed to enable sideways wheelchair transfers.

Accessories

Accessories improve comfort and tailor the basic wheelchair to individual needs and disability. A pump is routinely supplied, but a cushion, which improves comfort and minimises pressure sores,

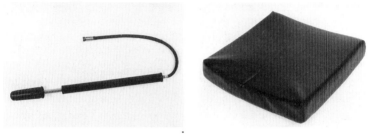

A pump *(left)* and cushion *(right)* should be regarded as essential accessories.

needs to be requested. Many types of cushion are available, but those made from 2 inch polyurethane foam with a polyvinylchloride cover are good for most purposes.[3] Foam deteriorates with use, however, and needs replacing after about two years. A plywood or chipfoam baseboard further improves the cushioning effect by eliminating seat sag. When a patient has a special problem—for example, if he is overweight, has previous ischial sores, or is a constant wheelchair user—specialist advice should be sought from the disablement service centre staff or a community occupational therapist.

Other common accessories include a detachable tray, desk sidearms (which allow closer positioning to a table), and a backrest cushion. A backrest extension is useful if the chair is to be used for long periods. Patients who have had a hemiplegic stroke often require a brake lever extension so that they can operate both brakes with the unaffected arm.

Home adaptations

Narrow doorways and steps which limit the free use of a wheelchair must be identified when the chair is ordered. Local authorities (hous-

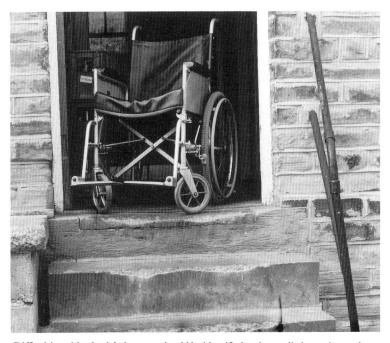

Difficulties with wheelchair access should be identified and remedied as an integral part of wheelchair prescription.

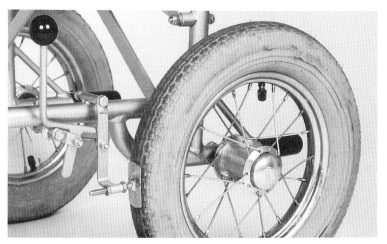

Wheelchair brakes operate by a metal plate being forced against the pneumatic tyre by a lever mechanism. For the brakes to function effectively it is therefore essential to keep the tyres fully inflated.

ing departments) will undertake home adaptations, usually on the advice of a community occupational therapist. Unfortunately it is often some months before the work is completed.

Follow up

Ensure that the chair has met the patient's requirements, and check that he knows how to use it safely. Disablement service centre chairs are supplied with a brief handbook, which describes the wheelchair, its use, and how to maintain it. However, some patients need additional instruction from the referring doctor or occupational therapist.[4] All wheelchair users should be trained to check the pneumatic tyres and brakes regularly. Repairs for disablement service centre chairs are carried out by an approved local repairer and those for privately purchased chairs are organised by the retailer.

Electric wheelchairs

Electric wheelchairs are heavy, are difficult to fold, and require space — for example, in a garage — for storage and battery recharging. Those available from the DHSS are provided only after assessment by artificial limb and appliance centre medical and technical staff. DHSS electric wheelchairs fall into two categories:

(1) *Indoor electric wheelchairs*, considered for patients who are unable to walk or use a manually self propelled chair and who are likely to gain independence from wheelchair mobility.

(2) *Outdoor electric wheelchairs*, which are controlled by an attendant and considered when the attendant is too weak to push a manual chair, or when the district is hilly.

Outdoor occupant controlled electric wheelchairs are not available through disablement service centres. This type of chair (and the other categories) may be purchased privately. Several firms provide these chairs, and various models are available. But they are expensive. If the patient receives the mobility allowance this can be used to obtain an electric wheelchair through the motability scheme.

1 Department of Health and Social Security. *Wheelchairs—a guide to clinical prescription*. DHSS Appliance Service, Warbreck Hill, Blackpool, Lancashire.
2 Department of Health and Social Security. *Handbook of wheelchairs (MHM 408)*. DHSS Security Store, Manchester Road, Heywood, Lancashire.
3 Jay P. *Wheelchair cushions summary report*. DHSS Security Store, Manchester Road, Heywood, Lancashire.
4 British Red Cross Society. *People in wheelchairs (hints for helpers)*. London: British Red Cross Society.

Choosing easy chairs for the disabled

MALCOLM ELLIS

Although good seating can contribute to the well being of the elderly and those with arthritis, who may spend long periods sitting, these people often have problems with their chairs.

When a person rises from a chair the forces in the knee joint are up to seven times body weight, a large force for painful joints to bear. Patients with muscle wasting and stiffness may have difficulty in rising; so may those with rheumatoid hands who experience pain when pushing or gripping and those whose shoulders cannot take the brunt of weight transfer. Obesity frequently supervenes because of inactivity, thereby compounding the problem of rising.

Seat height

The higher the seat the easier it is to rise from. The joint and muscle forces used in lifting from a high seat are 20% less than those required in rising from a low one. If the seat is too high, however, the feet may dangle, causing fatigue and discomfort, and the seat may indent the back of the thighs near the knee.

Seat angle

A horizontal seat with a sloping back rest is uncomfortable and causes the patient to slide forward. When the seat slope is too great rising from the chair is difficult. The seat should therefore slope gently backwards. An angle of 6° is a good compromise.

Seat construction

If the chair has a hard support rail at the front underneath the cushion the edge may dig into the thighs as the cushion sags, causing pain and restricting circulation. "Hammocking" of the seat often causes shear stresses on the buttocks, resulting in pain in the hips and possible pressure sores.

The cushion or seat should be made of good quality materials. Foams quickly lose their resilience, and the sitter then feels the hard bottom of the seat. The resultant high loads under the ischial tuberosities can lead to pressure sores. Foams and coverings should allow a flow of air through the seat to reduce the effects of perspiration and localised overheating of the skin. Open cell foams are therefore preferable to the closed cell variety.

Covers

Incontinent patients will be more comfortable if the seat covering can absorb moisture. Removable sheepskin covers are suitable as these feel soft and warm, can absorb a large amount of moisture yet still feel dry, and are easily washed. They also allow good ventilation, reducing localised overheating of the skin, and help absorb perspiration. Covers should be hard wearing, and the material should be neither too rough (which would restrict movement) nor too slippery. Sewn in buttons on the cushion or backrest can dig into the flesh and should be avoided.

Backrest

The human back is not straight but curved, with a cervical lordosis, thoracic kyphosis, and lumbar lordosis. The ideal backrest should be shaped accordingly, obviating the need for extra cushions, which may slip, become squashed, or be awkward to adjust.

If the backrest is too upright the muscles in the back tense to stop the trunk from falling forward, so relaxation is difficult. If it is inclined too greatly the body tends to slide down the chair and getting up is difficult. The backrest should slope gently backward and be high enough to support the full length of the back.

The head should also be supported. A protruding headrest should, however, be avoided as it pushes the head forward, forcing the neck muscles to restrain the head; this results in neck pain. Although wings on a chair are popular, care must be taken that they do not socially isolate the sitter.

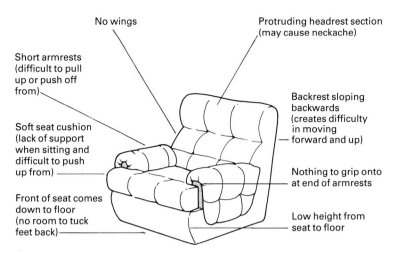

No wings

Protruding headrest section
(may cause neckache)

Short armrests
(difficult to pull
up or push off
from)

Soft seat cushion
(lack of support
when sitting and
difficult to push
up from)

Front of seat comes
down to floor
(no room to tuck
feet back)

Backrest sloping
backwards
(creates difficulty
in moving
forward and up)

Nothing to grip onto
at end of armrests

Low height from
seat to floor

A poor chair for a patient with arthritis.

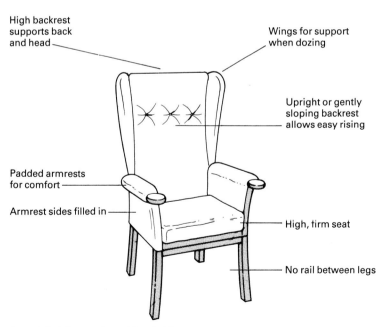

High backrest
supports back
and head

Wings for support
when dozing

Upright or gently
sloping backrest
allows easy rising

Padded armrests
for comfort

Armrest sides filled in

High, firm seat

No rail between legs

A good chair for a patient with arthritis.

Armrests

Armrests which are too low inhibit rising. Those which are too high cause people to hunch their shoulders when resting their arms on them. Armrests of the correct height greatly assist rising from the seated position. Biomechanical analysis has shown them to be of greater value than a high seat in minimising the joint and muscle forces used when rising.

Also, handgrips greatly assist in rising, especially initially. Large rounded ends will be less painful to grip for those with arthritic hands. Longer armrests facilitate rising more than short ones. For added comfort armrests should be partially padded. Filled in sides help retain warmth, exclude draughts, and prevent items such as newspapers, knitting, etc from falling from the chair. Filled in sides also retain fallen cigarettes, however, so a chair made from fire resistant materials is desirable.

General construction

Strength, stability, and safety are of great importance for the arthritic easy chair user. A chair which is high and has splayed legs has increased stability. The chair should be constructed so that the sitter can tuck his feet back under the seat: rising is easier when the body's centre of gravity falls over the ankles at an earlier point in the rising action.

Some people use their furniture as a support to aid walking within their home; others flop into their chairs heavily. Chairs should therefore be sturdy and well built.

The disabled are more at risk in a fire than the ambulant. Although manufacturers may argue against fireproofing of seating materials because of the extra cost, the Leeds survey[1] showed that arthritic people consider this to be quite a high priority when choosing a chair.

Castors may help in moving the chair, and larger castors may be better than smaller ones, which might sink into carpets. For those who flop into their chairs only the front legs should be fitted with castors.

Although function is paramount, patients should be pleased with the appearance of their chairs; otherwise they may not use them. The chair should fit in with existing furniture in size, design, and colour so that the disabled person does not feel unnecessarily different.

Attachments such as ashtrays, tables, crutch and stick holders, side pockets and footrests (for those with fixed flexion deformities) can be of great benefit for many disabled people.

Mechanised chairs

Patients who experience great difficulty in rising, even from a well designed chair, may benefit from a spring assisted seat (to be placed in their own easy chair), or a spring assisted chair. This may, however, be a compromise: some patients have commented that although a spring assisted seat helped them to rise, it was hard and uncomfortable to sit on. A motorised chair which lifts the patient into a standing position, or raises him to a higher seat level, may be the answer for those for whom rising from a chair is a severe problem. It is advisable to seek professional advice about the suitability and safety of these devices for a specific patient.

Further advice

Professional advice may be obtained from the local disabled living centre. An appointment is usually required to visit the centre, where a large number of suitable chairs (and other aids) can be tried and their merits discussed. Further information can be obtained from the Disabled Living Foundation, 380–384 Harrow Road, London W9 2HU (telephone 01 289 6111).

A pamphlet entitled *Are you sitting comfortably?* describes what to look for when choosing an easy chair. This publication is available from the Arthritis and Rheumatism Council, 41 Eagle Street, London WC1R 4AR.

A selection of easy chairs is available through social services departments. But it is such a limited selection that a patient may compromise by choosing a chair not entirely suitable for his needs, and which can be detrimental to him. It is recommended that the patient should contact his local community occupational therapist for guidance.

Finally, the best advice anyone can offer to someone choosing an easy chair is "try it before you buy it, preferably for as long as you can."

1 Ellis MI, Munton JS, Chamberlain MA. *Seating for the elderly and arthritic.* London: DHSS, 1983.

Aids for urinary incontinence

NIGEL SMITH

Urinary incontinence is common: an average general practice of 2500 patients will include at least 40 people of different ages with moderate or severe symptoms.[1] Common causes include constipation, diuretics, infection, and low fluid intake. Specialist urodynamic investigation is carried out by urologists and gynaecologists, and an increasing range of treatments for the unstable bladder and for pelvic floor weakness is provided by continence clinics staffed by nurse continence advisers working in conjunction with doctors.[2] Unfortunately, most people with urinary incontinence do not seek professional help; instead they attempt, with varying degrees of success, to conceal their symptoms by using sanitary towels or household materials such as strips of bed linen. Whatever the cause of incontinence it is essential to make the patient comfortable while investigations and treatment are carried out.

Design of incontinence pads and pants

Daytime incontinence in women is best controlled by an aid which is comfortable to wear, easy to use, highly absorbent, and discreet. Patients differ in the importance they attach to each design factor: some like an aid which is designed not to distort the contours of their figure; others give priority to absorbency and comfort. So it is important to offer the patient a choice. Additionally, the continence adviser should explain how each aid is used, because without professional advice it is easy for the patient to misunderstand the manufacturer's instructions.

Pads usually contain wood pulp overlain by a polyester cover stock and have a plastic backing. The cover stock allows urine through while keeping the patient's skin dry. The plastic backing overlaps the

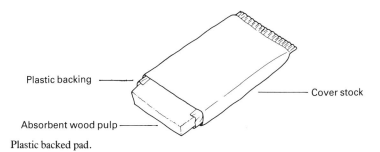

Plastic backing

Cover stock

Absorbent wood pulp

Plastic backed pad.

edges of the wood pulp to reduce leakage. Pads are normally changed at convenient times of day and the number of pads used has been shown to have little relation to absorbency. New substances such as highly absorbent gels have few advantages over conventional materials; although they are less bulky they are more expensive and do not "look" absorbent.

An extensive comparative study recently carried out by the DHSS[3] on the performance of various types of pads and pants concludes that three designs will suit the needs of most patients. Mild and moderate incontinence can be effectively controlled by a marsupial system such as the Kanga single pad used with Kanga lady pants, which are worn instead of normal underwear. A pad without backing fits into a waterproof pouch separated from the wearer by one way polyester material. The chief drawbacks of this system are that changing the

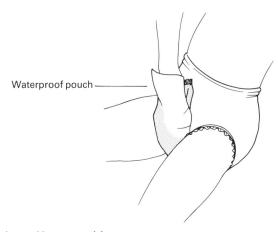

Waterproof pouch

Pad being inserted into marsupial pants.

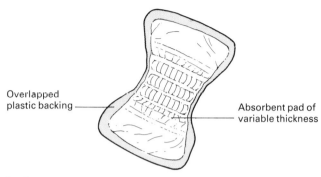

Overlapped plastic backing

Absorbent pad of variable thickness

Shaped pad.

pad requires some degree of dexterity and that patients with more severe symptoms experience problems of odour and are likely to get their hands wet when removing the used pad.

Severe day and night incontinence is best controlled by using a pad backed with plastic and worn with stretch pants. Pads designed to fit the body, such as the Mölnlycke Tenaform range, seem least affected by leakage and splitting of the cover stock.

The third option is the all in one diaper; it is similar in design to children's nappies and includes reusable tapes, one way cover stock, and elasticated legs. Designs such as Tenders are used in some longer stay institutions. Major drawbacks are the need for two or three changes per night and the unwillingness of patients to accept a nappy design.

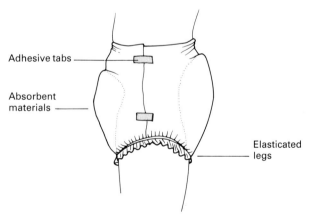

Adhesive tabs

Absorbent materials

Elasticated legs

All in one diaper.

External incontinence devices for men

For men there are two further options: a dribble pouch for mild symptoms and a penile sheath for moderate and severe symptoms. The dribble pouch is worn inside a normal pair of pants and held in place by an adhesive tab. Its limitations are that it absorbs only small amounts of urine and demands a close fit.

A penile sheath may be held in place by a strip of latex around the penis. The sheath drains into a leg bag, ideally with a textile backing and foam and velcro straps. Problems include skin erosion due to the adhesive strip or urine stasis, twisting of the sheath, penile retraction during voiding causing leakage, and skin abrasions associated with the leg bag and straps.

Incontinence sheets

Some people dislike wearing any system to contain incontinence, particularly at night. Plastic bed covers tend to cause excessive sweating and do little to reduce aroma. Multilayer incontinence sheets commonly end up crumpled at the bottom of the bed; and because they contain recycled paper there is a risk of transmitting clostridial organisms to skin ulcers. A rewashable absorbent sheet can be used with a plastic draw sheet to protect the mattress. The principal disadvantage is the cost: each patient needs three sheets—one in use, one in the wash, and one drying.

The provision of incontinence aids

Marsupial pads and pants, body shaped pads and stretch pants, adult diapers, and bed covers are available to community nurses through district and regional supplies officers. Penile sheaths can be prescribed by FP10, but dribble pouches and Kylie sheets must be bought. The Association of Continence Advisors' directory summarises the full range of incontinence products available in the United Kingdom.[4]

If there were more feedback from users and community nurses to supplies departments designs that are cost effective could more readily be identified and the supplies system thereby improved. Since the materials and characteristics of incontinence aids that are worn are continually being changed and improved there is a constant need for clinical trials comparing the performance of different pads. Reordering supplies could be simplified by using either a card index or a computerised system, and a facilitator could stock and update a demonstration case of available pads and pants.

Financial assistance to offset the cost of incontinence may be obtained through (a) attendance allowance; (b) invalid care allowance; (c) supplementary benefit—extra laundry addition, regular baths, need for attendance, special wear and tear on clothing.[5]

Laundry services

A "black bag" collection system may be available through the environmental health department or area health authority; laundry services are available through the area social services department. Both facilities are free of charge.

I wish to thank the Department of Health and Social Security for permission to adapt Crown Copyright illustrations from *Incontinence garments: results of a DHSS study*.

1 McGrother CW, Castleden CM, Duffin H, Clarke M. Provision of services of incontinent elderly people at home. *J Epidemiol Comm Health* 1986;40:134–8.
2 Norton C. *Nursing for continence*. Beaconsfield, Bucks. Beaconsfield Publishers, 1986.
3 Department of Health and Social Security. Incontinence garments: results of a DHSS study. *Health Equipment Information*, 1986;159.
4 Association of Continence Advisors. *Directory of continence aids and appliances*, 4th edn. London: Association of Continence Advisors, 1988.
5 Continence Advisory Service. *Financial benefits for people with problems of incontinence*. Newcastle upon Tyne: Newcastle upon Tyne Council for the Disabled, 1987.

Urinary catheters

P W BELFIELD

Catheters are used in urological surgery and when other methods of managing urinary incontinence fail. Ten per cent of hospital patients receive an indwelling urinary catheter at some time during their admission,[1] and the use of such catheters results in a significant morbidity and mortality.[2-4]

Which catheter should be used?

Urinary catheters should be carefully chosen for each patient, with particular regard to the duration of catheterisation. Important factors are the material used, the diameter, the balloon volume, and the sex of the patient. Also, the correct drainage bag system should be used.

Material

Catheters are made of plastic, latex, teflon, or silicone. Plastic and latex catheters are suitable for the measurement of residual volumes. Latex is commonly associated with encrustation of protein and salts on the catheter and in longer term use can cause urethral strictures. Silicone and teflon coated or pure silicone catheters do not irritate the urethra; this allows them to remain in situ for long periods (up to 2–3 months). Latex catheters are cheaper (about 50p each) than silicone and teflon coated or pure silicone catheters (about £3·50 each).

Diameter

Catheter diameter is measured in French gauge or Charrière size (1 Ch = 0·33 mm = external diameter of catheter shaft). A wide range of sizes is available. The catheter selected should be the smallest capable of giving adequate drainage while providing maximum comfort to the patient. Problems tend to occur with larger sizes; so the common practice of changing to catheters of wider diameter to prevent leaking around the instrument (bypassing) is ill advised.[5]

Balloon volume

Two balloon volumes are commonly available: 5 ml and 20–30 ml. Larger balloons are useful postoperatively and occasionally in chronically catheterised women who have weak pelvic musculature, but they tend to irritate the bladder and cause bypassing. Balloons should be inflated with sterile water, not saline (which crystallises in the inflation channel, thus preventing deflation) or air (which causes the balloon to float on the surface of the urine). Remember that 5 ml of water will underinflate a 5 ml balloon because some water is "lost" along the length of the catheter. To ensure even inflation use 7–10 ml of sterile water. To avoid urethral trauma and pain on deflation allow several minutes for the balloon to drain before withdrawing the catheter.

Sex of patient

Many doctors and nurses are unaware that shorter length catheters are available for women. These are 21 cm long, whereas the standard length is 40–45 cm; they obviate the use of unsightly external tubing.

Drainage bag systems

Only use large volume (1–2 l) surgical drainage bags during the period immediately after an operation. Leg bags and other drainage bag systems—for example, pants with pouches to hold the bag—can be discreetly hidden from sight yet readily accessible for emptying.[6] These systems help to maintain the dignity and morale of the patient.

Problems of urinary catheterisation

Leakage and blockage

Leakage can occur when a catheter is too wide or has a large balloon. Encrustation causes blockage and leakage. Bypassing is also caused by involuntary bladder contractions, which may be diminished by administering bladder stabilising drugs such as imipramine. These problems are aggravated by the easily treatable problem of faecal impaction.

Infection

Patients with long term indwelling catheters inevitably have bacteria in the urine. In these patients antibiotics should be reserved for symptomatic, febrile infections; otherwise their use produces a

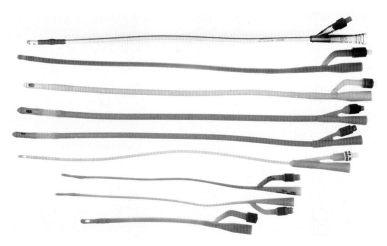

Wide range of catheter sizes.

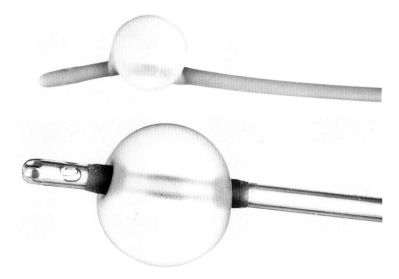

Balloons: 5 ml *(above)* and 30 ml *(below)*.

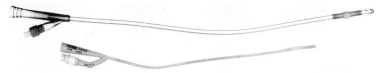

Short catheter for women.

change in bacterial flora with the potential for producing resistance. The addition of antibacterial substances to drainage bags is not effective in preventing bacteriuria.[1] From the few clinical trials so far carried out it seems that the use of washouts is also ineffective in this respect.

Catheter rejection

Instances of catheters being pushed out, pulled out, or falling out usually occur in frail, immobile, demented old people and accounts for 45% of all catheter changes in elderly inpatients.[3] Catheter rejection has a significant morbidity and mortality. Catheters which are seen to have been pulled out should not be replaced; instead, alternative methods for controlling incontinence should be used.[7] When the catheter is forcibly pushed out by an involuntary bladder contraction bladder stabilising drugs may be helpful. When catheters fall out owing to urethral dilatation from repeated catheterisation or pelvic floor laxity larger balloon volumes should be tried.

Failure of balloon deflation

The catheter cannot be removed when the balloon fails to deflate. Several methods have been devised for overcoming this problem — for example, introducing chloroform to dissolve the balloon and suprapubic percutaneous puncture — but none of these is ideal. The safest and most effective method is the introduction of a ureteric catheter stylet along the inflation channel.[8]

Physical and psychological difficulties

Embarrassment and loss of self esteem are common. Many patients are catheterised without the doctor's taking time to explain why a catheter is needed, how it works, and how long it will be in place. Catheter insertion and removal can be painful — so much so, in fact, that patients dread their next catheter change. These problems are often neglected.

Care of the chronically catheterised patient

Aim for better care by choosing the right catheter for each patient. Use small diameter catheters (12–16 Ch); small balloon volumes (5 ml); short catheters for women; drainage systems which do not offend the patient's dignity and which avoid traction on the catheter — for example, pants with pouches to hold the bag.

Ensure good fluid intake, as this provides the "best" bladder wash-out.

If there are no problems avoid "routine" changes. Doctors and nurses should regularly discuss problems and document each catheter change.

Booklets on urinary catheterisation, for both health workers and patients, are produced by catheter manufacturers such as Bard Ltd.

Most health districts now have specialist continence advisers, who are nurses. They have an important role in education and problem solving.

Urinary catheterisation should not be undertaken lightly. It offends dignity and can be painful, or even fatal. When it is essential care should be taken to choose the correct catheter and to prevent or treat problems to maintain the comfort and well being of the patient.

1 Kunin CM. The drainage bag additive saga. *Infect Contr* 1985;**6**:261–2.
2 Merguerian PA, Erturk E, Hulbert WC, *et al*. Peritonitis and abdominal free air due to intraperitoneal bladder perforation associated with indwelling urethral catheter drainage. *J Urol* 1985;**134**:747–50.
3 Belfield PW, Young JB, Mulley GP. Rejection of catheters. *Br Med J* 1985;**291**:108–9.
4 Macfarlane DE. Prevention and treatment of catheter-associated urinary tract infections. *J Infect* 1985;**10**:96–106.
5 Kennedy AP, Brocklehurst JC, Lye MDW. Factors related to the problems of long-term catheterization. *J Adv Nurs* 1983;**8**:207–12.
6 Kennedy AP. Nursing and the incontinent patient. In: Brocklehurst JC, ed. *Urology in the elderly*. London: Churchill Livingstone, 1984.
7 Castleden CM, Duffin HM. Guidelines for controlling urinary incontinence without drugs or catheters. *Age Ageing* 1981;**10**:186–90.
8 Browning GGP, Barr L, Horsburgh AG. Management of obstructed balloon catheters. *Br Med J* 1984;**289**:89–91.

Toilet aids

N D PENN

Toilet aids help to preserve the dignity and independence of a disabled person and may be crucial in enabling him or her to continue living at home. The commonest difficulties experienced by the disabled are getting to the lavatory and rising from the toilet seat.[1] There are aids designed to overcome these problems.

Commodes and urinals

If a person cannot reach the toilet because of difficulty with mobility or access—for example, the toilet is upstairs or outside—a commode should be considered. The many commodes available are based on three designs: stool or armchair commodes and chemical toilets.

Stool commodes have no arm or back rests and thus offer no support to the user, who must therefore have good balance and be able to stand unaided. They are, however, smaller and less obtrusive than the alternatives.

Armchair commodes may be of tubular metal, wood, or artificial cane construction. Commodes made from wood or artificial cane are generally of fixed height (although some manufacturers offer the same model in different heights) and do not have detachable arms. They resemble pieces of household furniture. The tubular metal commodes, although more conspicuous, are more versatile. A commode should be the right height for the user, and some commodes are available with adjustable seats and arm rests. The arms may also be removed to make it easier to transfer the patient to the commode from bed or wheelchair. The commode should also be of a suitable width; and for stability the base should be wider than the arms. Some models have wheels or castors so they can be easily pushed, but they are designed not to move when in use. Folding commodes are available for transport in cars. Remember that an oval aperture is preferable, especially for men who might otherwise miss the pan.

Although commodes are intended to maintain independence, the users inevitably depend on others—usually family or friends—to empty and clean them. Through embarrassment some users attempt to empty the commode themselves. A round or oval steel bowl is easier to clean than one shaped like a bed pan (which has a rim to prevent spillage); furthermore, the contents can be more easily emptied into the lavatory. A neutralising agent such as Nilodor reduces the odour.

Commodes may be borrowed from the local health authority at the request of the general practitioner or district nurse. These are usually of a basic design with few additional features. Commodes may also be borrowed from charitable organisations, and a wider choice is available privately.

Chemical toilets should be considered in cases where commodes cannot be emptied regularly. The models available range from modified commodes to variations of the conventional toilets used for camping or in aeroplanes. In general the conventional designs tend to be too low for the disabled. Some manufacturers sell frames which lift the toilet to a suitable height; alternatively, a standard toilet frame can be used. However, certain models are designed so that the height can be adjusted. When choosing a toilet the height of the seat, accessibility of the flush handle, position of the arm rests, and overall stability should be considered. Capacity is also a factor: the greater the capacity the more often the toilet can be used before it is emptied, but the task of emptying it becomes harder as the weight increases.

If there is a genuine need chemical toilets can be obtained at the request of the general practitioner or district nurse from the local health authority. Alternatively, they can be bought from camping shops. If the toilet is obtained from the local authority an arrangement will be made to empty it on a regular basis; if it is obtained elsewhere private arrangements may have to be made. The local authority provides the first batch of chemical fluid with a toilet it has supplied; thereafter, the user must provide his own. As the substance is only available from camping centres this may prove difficult.

A person may use a urinal at night instead of getting out of bed to use a commode or the lavatory. Some urinals for men are designed to be unspillable, or can be made so by the insertion of a non-spill adaptor. Those for women include the slipper pan and suba seal. A urinal can be used by a patient in a wheelchair if a split cushion has been fitted. Some chairs have a drainage system installed for those for

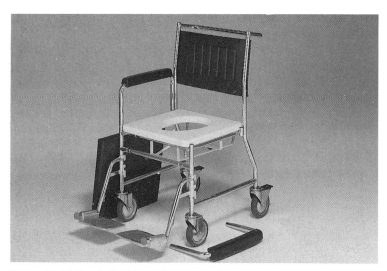

Commode with detachable side arm for easy transfer. (Courtesy of Carters (J & A) Ltd.)

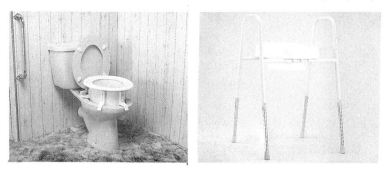

Adjustable raised toilet seat *(left)*; free standing, adjustable toilet frame *(right)*. Courtesy of Carters (J & A) Ltd.)

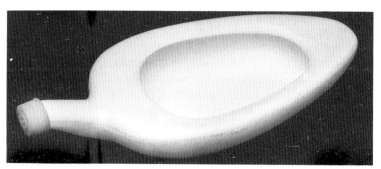

Suba seal.

whom emptying the urinal is a problem. In general, however, urinals are difficult to use and rarely completely successful.

Raised toilet seats

Disabled people—particularly those with severe arthritis of the knees and hips—who have difficulty rising from a chair are likely to have trouble getting off a normal toilet, the height of which ranges from 350 to 400 mm. Carpeting the floor or providing foot stops or slip resistant strips may help them to stand by providing a better purchase for their feet.

If the toilet seat must be raised permanently the whole toilet can be set on blocks or, alternatively, a new purpose built toilet can be installed. But a raised toilet seat, although more conspicuous, is less expensive and more practical than either of these options. All toilet seats fit directly on to the pan; they are unstable if fitted on to the seat. A lightweight, easily fitted raised seat is important if a disabled person has to lift it on and off, but once in place it should be secure and must not damage the pan. A convex seat is more comfortable than a concave one; and a matt finish prevents adherence to the skin. A long aperture helps to facilitate personal cleansing. The height of the seat has to be assessed for each user. This is best done by trial and error at home. Most people's needs can be met by choosing one of five seat heights (450, 475, 500, 525, and 550 mm).[2] Some seats are made with a means of adjusting the height; they can also be adjusted to fit different sizes of pan.

Toilet rails

Those who are unsteady on their feet may be helped by the presence of suitably positioned toilet rails. Any grab rail must be firmly enough attached to take the strain of a person's weight. A horizontal rail at waist level provides support when the patient walks into the room, when he manipulates his clothes, and when standing and sitting. If the user has function in only one arm rails will need to be installed on both sides of the room. Hinged horizontal rails are available; these may be folded away when not in use.

Neither sloping nor vertical rails have been shown to be as effective as horizontal ones in providing support for someone getting on and off the toilet.[2]

Toilet frames

Floor standing frames built to fit round the lavatory provide as much support as horizontal rails and can be used when the latter are impracticable. Such frames can be free standing, fixed to the floor, or attached to the back of the pan. Fixed frames are better than free standing ones, particularly when pressure is exerted on one side only, as by a patient with hemiplegia. However, if a person can balance and his coordination is good a free standing frame should be considered, especially for those who want to take their frames with them when visiting relatives or friends. Some frames incorporate a built in raised toilet seat.

Wheelchairs

The wheelchair must be small enough to go through the doorway (in older houses the toilet entrance is often the narrowest). Ideally, there should be enough space for the user to manoeuvre the wheelchair to the side of the toilet. A combined bathroom and toilet is therefore preferable. Rehanging the door so that it opens outwards will provide more space and facilitate any rescue operation. The seat of the wheelchair and the seat of the toilet should be of more or less the same height for ease of transfer; a sliding board may be useful. If there is not enough space for the wheelchair to be positioned next to the toilet the user may have to approach the toilet seat from the front and, by using suitably positioned grab rails, swivel round on to it. Alternatively, he may transfer himself without swivelling, so that he is sitting back to front. Some people, particularly paraplegics and tetraplegics, prefer to transfer backwards. There are special wheelchair backrests available to make this possible.

A range of urinals is made for use in a wheelchair.

Provision of aids

Toilet aids can be obtained from social services, borrowed from local health authorities and certain charities (such as the British Red Cross), or bought privately.

Before an aid is provided an assessment should be carried out in the patient's home by an occupational therapist to decide which aid will be most effective. Adequate instruction in the use of the aid selected should be given and follow up visits made to ensure it is being used and maintained correctly. Any change in the condition or requirements of the disabled person can be assessed at these visits and any unused aids retrieved.

1 Chamberlain MA, Thornley G, Wright V. Evaluation of aids and equipment for bath and toilet. *Rheumatol Rehabil* 1978;**17**:187.
2 Page M, Cooper S, Feeney R. *The selection of toilet aids for disabled people.* Loughborough: Institute for Consumer Ergonomics, University of Technology.

Equipment for Bathing

J GEORGE, A A J KERR

Difficulty in bathing may occur with many neurological, orthopaedic, and medical conditions and is a problem for nearly half of all people aged over 75.[1] Bath aids should be considered for all those who would like help, in particular patients with severe arthritis affecting their hips and knees, those who have had strokes, and those with multiple sclerosis or Parkinson's disease.

Recommending a bath aid

Before recommending a bath aid it is essential to check that the patient has good access to the bathroom and is capable of using the aid correctly and safely. Patients must have enough strength in their arms to wash and dry themselves. The medical diagnosis is important as patients may improve or deteriorate, necessitating a regular review of the need for a particular aid.

Provision

General practitioners should refer patients who have difficulty in bathing to occupational therapists, based in social services departments or in hospital. In some districts, however, provision of bath aids can be arranged through district nurses. Assessment is carried out in the patient's own home and instructions are given on the correct use of the aid supplied. Ideally, the use and usefulness of a bath aid should be re-evaluated at regular intervals. Bath aids are also obtainable privately and on loan from certain charitable organisations, such as the British Red Cross.

Other considerations

Elderly people living alone who have problems with bathing should always make certain that someone else—for example, a daughter or a home help—is in the house when they take a bath, and they should leave the bathroom door unlocked. Patients with portable alarms should be reminded that the alarm must be removed before they get into the bath.

If bath aids are unlikely to be of help then there are alternatives: these include bathing at home with the help of a district nurse or bath attendant; bathing at a day centre or day hospital; having a strip wash or a shower. Nearly 10% of home visits by district nurses are to help with bathing.[2]

Mats

The upper side of a bath mat should be textured so that it provides a safe non-slip surface. The surface of the bath should be moistened and the mat pressed down to fix it firmly to the floor of the bath before the water is turned on. Bath mats tend to decay after about two years and should therefore be renewed regularly.

Boards

A bath board is useful for people who have difficulty in getting over the side of the bath. While sitting on the board a person can wash himself with the water in the bath, or he can sit under the shower. Bath boards have another useful function: they can be used as a perch from which the bather can ease himself down on to a bath seat or the floor of the bath. The board must be the right width for the bath, its surface should not be slippery when wet, it should allow easy transfer, and there should be no sharp edges. A bath board should be strong enough to bear the weight of the user.

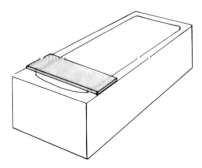

Bath board.

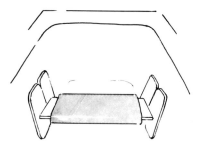

Bath seat.

Seats

Bath seats are designed for those who are unable to sit on the floor of the bath or at least to move to that position from any appreciable height. Either the user takes his bath sitting on the seat or he moves from the seat to the floor of the bath, washes himself, then returns to the seat before getting out of the bath. Rim suspended seats should be chosen for acrylic baths because seats with hinged support legs may puncture the walls of the bath. Bath seats are often used in conjunction with bath boards.

Rails

Bath rails are used to help a person get in and out of the bath or to help him manoeuvre once he is in the bath. There are three main types:

(*a*) tap rails, which are widely used but restrict movement in the bath;

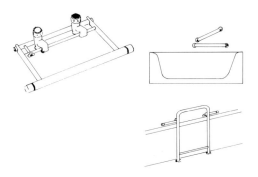

Bath rails.

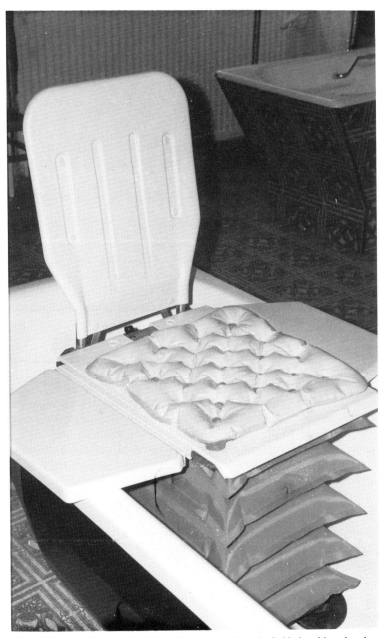

Mangar Booster inflated and positioned in the bath. Note the SuMed cushion placed on the seat. (Courtesy of Mangar Aids Ltd.)

(b) wall mounted rails, which should be fixed to the wall and positioned to suit the user;

(c) rim rails, which are fixed to the floor and secured to the edge of the bath.

All rails should be checked regularly to ensure that they are secure.

Other bath aids

There is a wide variety of other helpful bath aids, including:

(a) slatted bath boards, which allow the patient to shower while sitting;

(b) extended bathboards, which help the patient to get into the bath;

(c) bath seats which are moulded for greater security;

(d) bath inserts, which decrease the depth of the bath;

(e) inflatable bath seats, which can be lowered into the bath;

(f) hydraulic bath seats, which can be lowered into the bath and help the patient to get in;

(g) mechanical bath lifts, which can be lowered into the bath and help the patient to get in.

Effectiveness

Bath aids are effective in enabling disabled people to bathe.[3] To be most effective, however, they should be supplied only after the patient has been properly assessed and instructed in their use by an occupational therapist. In a survey of 140 people aged over 75 in a general practice we found that over 80% of the bath aids provided were used regularly but that there was an unmet need for aids in about 20% of the people assessed.[4]

1 Clark M, Clark S, Odell A, Jagger C. The elderly at home: health and social status. *Health Trends* 1984;**16**:3–7.

2 Ritchie J, Jacoby A, Bone M. *Access to primary health care*. London: HMSO, 1981.

3 Chamberlain MA, Thornely G, Stowe J, Wright V. Evaluation of aids and equipment for the bath II. A possible solution to the problem. *Rheumatol Rehabil* 1981;**20**:38–43.

4 George J, Binns VE, Clayden AD, Mulley GP. Aids and adaptations for the elderly at home: underprovided, underused, and undermaintained. *Br Med J* 1988;**296**:1365–6.

Hoists

KAREN WATERS

In some cases it can become difficult to move elderly or disabled people manually from bed to chair, from wheelchair to toilet, or in and out of a bath or car. A hoist can often ease the problem; it also reduces the risk of back injuries to nurses and other carers. "A hoist is a mechanical lifting aid designed to transport or lift someone from one place to another by means of suitable slings or a static seat."[1]

With over 40 different hoists available on the British market it is often difficult to select the most suitable one, and there may be occasions when other means will suffice.

(1) Transfers are always easier when surfaces are the same height: thus beds or chairs may be raised or lowered, or a raised toilet seat may be used.

(2) In some situations transfer boards may be sufficient.

(3) A monkey pole or grab rails may enable a disabled person who is confined to bed to achieve some independence.

(4) Alternative aids or appliances should be considered: for a person who is wheelchair bound the use of a U shaped cushion and a suitable urinal may mean that he will less often need to transfer to a toilet.

Who needs a hoist?

The potential hoist user may be anyone who suffers from a disability resulting from progressive disease, age, obesity, or a mixture of these conditions. Patients with multiple sclerosis are the largest group of hoist users.[2] Hoists should also be considered for those with muscular dystrophy, rheumatoid disease, stroke, cerebral palsy, and polio. Most people wish to maintain their independence and may find the use of a hoist invaluable.

Assessment

Detailed assessment is usually carried out by hospital or community occupational therapists, but in some places this may be done by physiotherapists or district nurses. The success of a hoist depends on the assessor's initial approach and the motivation of the user.

Points to be taken into account

- The diagnosis and the progress of the patient's condition
- Whether a hoist is acceptable to both the disabled person and the family
- Areas of transfer that are causing problems
- The home environment
- How much help with the hoist the patient is likely to obtain from his family and the community
- The physical fitness and strength of the carer or carers.

Training and practice

Training and supervision in the correct use of hoists and slings is vital. So is practice: it ensures that those concerned become familiar with the equipment and competent in its use. Problems arising during the daily routine should be identified at an early stage and practice modified to resolve the difficulties.

Follow up ensures the hoist is being used fully and that further problems have not arisen. If the person's condition is deteriorating then reassessment may be necessary and an alternative hoist or sling, or both, may need to be considered.

Mobile hoists

Mobile hoists range from small domestic models to larger models designed for use in hospitals and residential homes. They can be operated by hydraulic, electric, or hand wound screw mechanisms.

The smaller models can lift up to 20 stone (127 kg) and the larger ones up to 35 stone (220 kg). For manoeuvrability, castors are attached to the chassis. Large castors make it easier to move the hoist over carpets and across thresholds; however, they need greater clearance under a bed or bath. The chassis can be adjustable or fixed, depending on the type of hoist.

All models can span a standard size wheelchair. They can be

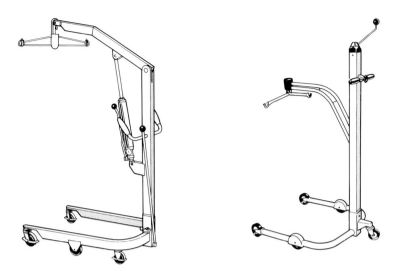

Hydraulic mobile hoist (*left*); Hand wound screw mechanism (*right*).

dismantled easily and transported, and this can be an advantage if the disabled person goes on holiday. The cost of a mobile hoist can range from £280 to £1020.

Fixed floor hoists

Hoists that are fixed to the floor are mainly used for getting someone in and out of a bath. They are useful also when space is limited. Most models can be operated only by helpers, but some are designed to be operated by either the user or the carer. The lifting capacity of a bath hoist is similar to that of a small mobile hoist. Prices range from £300 to £700.

Electric hoists may be attached permanently to an overhead gantry. If this is done transfers are, of course, limited to a fixed location. A more versatile arrangement can be provided by a straight or curved overhead track, which can, if desired, travel from one room to another. The tracking is attached to the ceiling joists. A spreader bar with sling attachments is fixed to the lower end of a spool of tape which then fits into the motor box. The bar is controlled by two pull cords, which simply enables the user to be raised or lowered. In more sophisticated models pull cords permit sideways movement.

These hoists must be installed by the manufacturer or by someone who is experienced in this type of work.

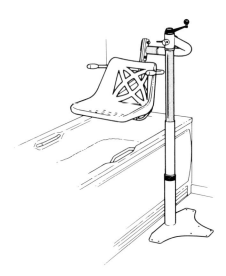

Autolift.

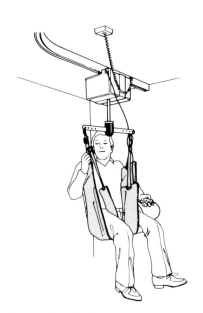

An electric hoist fitted to an overhead track.

An electric hoist should be considered if the following apply:
- The helper may not be strong enough to push a portable hoist
- There is adequate space
- The disabled person is able to take the sling on and off and is likely to become more independent than he would with another type of hoist
- The home is structurally suitable
- Funds are available to meet the cost, which can be over £1000.

Car hoists

Getting in and out of a car can be difficult for some disabled people. A hoist, operated by a hydraulic mechanism, can be fixed to the car roof by steel clamps, but it can only be operated by a helper. Some mobile hoists can be used to transfer a person from a wheelchair into a car, but this operation only works when the ground is flat and there are no kerbs. Car hoists should not be confused with wheelchair lifting devices attached to the car, which are useful only for the disabled person who is able independently to transfer himself into a car. The lifting capacity of a car hoist is up to 95 kg, and prices can vary from £200 to £500.

Maintenance of hoists

It is vital to maintain a hoist and check its load capacity yearly. Following the guarantee period, maintenance contracts can be negotiated with the manufacturer or a qualified engineer. Ideally, a contract should include a 24 hour repair service. Prices, however, may vary.

Slings

Slings are made in a variety of sizes, styles, and materials. The various fabrics—which include nylon weave, polyester, and terylene—are all washable and rot proof. In one major survey of hoists it was noted that nearly two thirds of slings were made of nylon.[1]

Because slings are difficult to remove some people sit in them all day.[2] Slings can be either fully or partly lined with synthetic sheepskin to avoid the risk of pressure sores. Care should be taken to ensure that the material does not fray as slings with damaged edges can prove

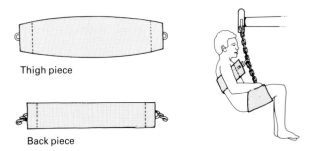

Thigh piece

Back piece

Band sling.

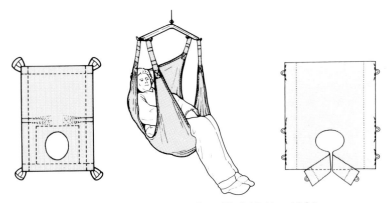

All in one hammock sling (*left*); hammock sling with divided legs (*right*).

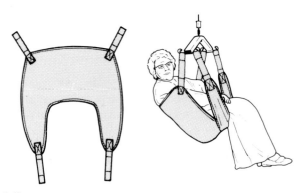

Universal sling.

dangerous. Alterations must be carried out by the manufacturer: they should never be done on a domestic sewing machine.

A sufficiently wide range of slings is available to meet most people's needs, but specially designed slings can be ordered if none of the standard ones is suitable. Ideally the user should be given a minimum of three slings — one in use, one in the wash, and one spare in case of soiling or damage.

It is important that the sling should be one recommended by the manufacturer of the hoist. The use of a different sling may invalidate the manufacturer's guarantee.

Attachments

Slings can be attached to hoists either by chains or loops. Loop attachments are made from webbing straps and are fixed at two points. They are simple, less noisy, and easier to use than chains. Chains, however, give a greater choice of suspension, offering more variation in the portions that can be adopted and hence increased comfort.

Band sling

This sling consists of two separate bands, attached by chains. One band goes round the back and chest and the other round the thighs. The arms must always be *outside* the upper strip; otherwise the patient will slip straight down through the sling. Band slings are suitable for people who are not seriously disabled — those who may be able to use the device without the help of a carer.

They are, however, unsuitable for (*a*) the more severely disabled person who may be suffering from muscle weakness, paralysis, or severe spasms, for he or she may slip through the back and thigh pieces; (*b*) a person whose shoulder joints are painful, for he may find the band slings pull on these joints; (*c*) the confused patient, because he may be unstable in these slings.

Hammock sling

The all in one sling can help the more severely disabled person. It gives support to the trunk, pelvis, and thighs and may incorporate a commode aperture.

The hammock sling with divided legs provides separate support for each thigh and enables the sling easily to be removed and repositioned under the user. It also has the advantage that users who are in wheelchairs do not need to sit in the sling all day. The incorporation of a commode aperture has obvious advantages.

Universal sling

This is easy and quick to use and is often issued as a standard sling. It includes a toilet aperture.

Supply

In some hospitals wards are equipped with a mobile or electric hoist. In others therapy departments may have a limited supply of hoists, which can be loaned to wards or used for assessment. A range of hoists is available in each health district for training purposes.

The health authority's home loans equipment service may have a small stock of mobile hoists available on temporary loan. When a person who needs a hoist is to be discharged home from hospital this service should be considered. The provision of the more common hoist and universal sling for long term use is normally through the social services department. When a more specialised hoist or sling is necessary social services may have to consider the cost implication.

The time taken to supply these aids varies from district to district, with inordinate delays occurring in certain areas; sometimes, too, the hoist provided is not the one requested.[2] Occasionally a charity such as the League of Friends, Round Table, or Rotary Club, may help in providing a hoist.

Before he buys a hoist privately a patient should seek the advice of a qualified person not connected with the manufacturer and insist that the hoist is demonstrated in the environment in which it is to be used.

A well maintained hoist is rarely the cause of an accident. Accidents usually occur through misuse, incorrect assessments, or inappropriate fittings. Some community services are so acutely concerned about these avoidable accident risks that they limit their hoist and sling provision to a very narrow range.

Conclusion

A hoist is a valuable aid for carers when lifting a heavy or disabled person becomes difficult. But hoists are expensive, occupy a lot of space, and may initially cause anxiety to patient and carer. Hoists should therefore only be provided when alternative strategies (lifting techniques, other equipment) have been considered.

The role of the occupational therapist in assessment and training is crucial. Only by careful assessment of the patient, family, and home environment can the appropriate hoist and sling be chosen; only by careful instruction can users overcome their fears of hoists and become confident and competent in their use.

1 Tarling C. *Hoists and their use*. London: Heinemann, 1980.
2 Haworth RJ, Nichols PJR. Hoists in the home: their recommendation and use. *Rheum Rehabil* 1980;**19**:42–51.

Appendix

Other sources of information

- *Hoists and their Use* by Christine Tarling (Heinemann, 1980) was published in response to a growing awareness that the problems of assessment and of prescribing hoists had received only minor coverage and information for both individual as well as professional users was hard to find.
- *The Equipment for the Disabled* series includes a booklet entitled *Hoists and Lifts*. This publication provides a comprehensive list of aids for the disabled and is compiled by the Nuffield Orthopaedic Centre, Mary Marlborough Lodge, Headington, Oxford OX3 7LD.
- The Disabled Living Foundation, 380 Harrow Road, London W9 2HU, publishes up to date lists of equipment, in which hoists are included. The names and addresses of manufacturers are given. It also issues relevant publications, such as *Choosing a Hoist*, and provides other useful information.
- Twice a year a large exhibition, NAIDEX, shows equipment for the disabled and the elderly. It is a useful visual and practical source of information as many companies attend with displays of old and new products.
- Information about hoists can also be obtained from disabled living centres and demonstration centres throughout the country.

Artificial limbs

DUNCAN H G COTTER

In 1986 there were 5596 new referrals for artificial limbs in England, Wales, and Northern Ireland. Artificial limbs not only improve the mobility or manipulative ability of someone who has lost a limb but also restore his self image. A patient who lacks the whole or part of an arm or leg should be considered for a prosthesis (artificial replacement), given that he has the physical and intellectual capacity to use one.

Referrals for artificial limbs in England, Wales, and Northern Ireland, 1986

Reason for amputation	Leg	Arm
Vascular insufficiency	3447	14
Diabetes	1064	2
Trauma	383	138
Malignancy	189	31
Congenital	36	93
Others	190	9

Artificial limbs are provided free to war pensioners and to patients who are eligible for National Health Service treatment. The service is provided by regional disablement service centres. The loss of a leg is much more common than the loss of an arm. It tends to occur in older people, usually as a result of vascular insufficiency or diabetes.

Assessment

Artificial limbs are more often underused than misused and so detailed assessment is important. If an artificial limb is to be successful not only must the patient want it but it must offer advantages over the alternatives—for example, for someone who has lost a leg a

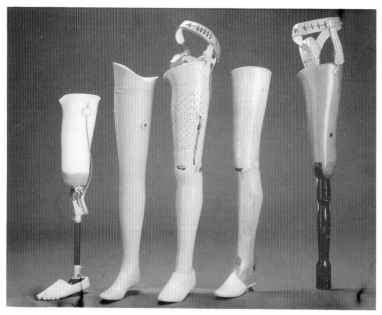

Development of above knee artificial limbs from the peg leg *(far right)* to modern modular construction *(far left)*. (Courtesy of J E Hanger & Co Ltd.)

wheelchair may offer as much mobility as a prosthesis. The doctor must ensure that the patient is able to put on and take off the prosthesis, or that carers are available to do this. He must make certain that a patient has enough cardiorespiratory reserve to cope with the increased energy demands of walking with an artificial leg.

Types of prosthesis

The design of an artificial leg is determined by the level of loss, which ranges from partial foot loss to total limb ablation by hindquarter amputation. Most commonly legs are amputated above the knee or below the knee.

Above knee prosthesis

The upper part is a socket specially contoured to fit on to the patient's residual limb (stump). The weight of the body is transmitted by the ischial tuberosity on to a seating that forms part of the socket. Attached to the socket is a suspension system to hold the prosthesis in

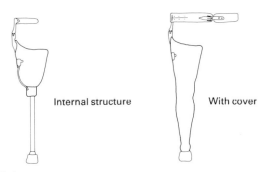

Internal structure   With cover

Above knee limb.

place and guide its movement. Below the socket is a knee mechanism to allow flexion when the patient sits down. Some knee mechanisms are designed to allow movement when the patient walks, others lock to give secure support. A metal or plastic shin joins the knee to an ankle and foot unit.

Below knee prosthesis

The Patella tendon bearing prosthesis is the one most commonly used today. The residual limb fits into a socket, which is shaped to distribute the weight of the body over pressure tolerant areas of skin below the knee joint while allowing the joint to function. There is a resilient foam liner between the residual limb and the rigid socket. Pressure must be avoided over bony prominences and the distal end of the residual limb by allowing extra clearance. Below the socket the limb is similar to the above the knee limb. The prosthesis is held in place by a strap above the knee, an elastic stocking, or shaped extensions of the socket which grip the femoral condyles.

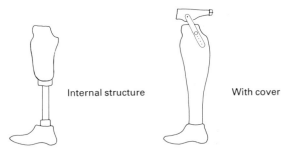

Internal structure   With cover

Below knee limb.

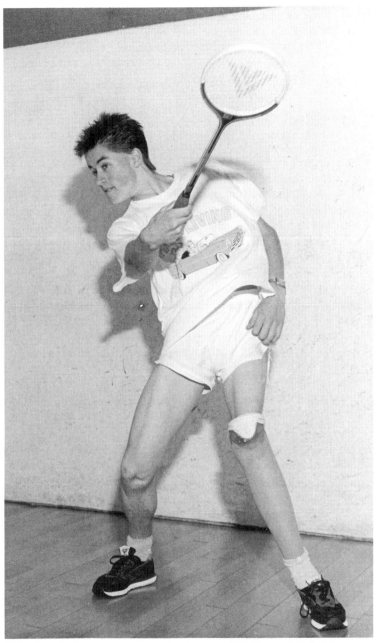

Below knee limb wearer playing squash. (Courtesy of J E Hanger & Co Ltd.)

Most leg prostheses are functional, but a small number are purely for cosmetic use by patients in wheelchairs.

Except in cases of limited partial hand loss, arm prostheses are available as either functional limbs or limbs that are primarily cosmetic.

Training and follow up

Artificial limb wearers need careful instruction in the use of their prosthesis and may need further help if specific problems arise or changes are made to the prescription. Gait training and instruction with leg prostheses are given by physiotherapists, usually at a local hospital. Training in the use of arm prostheses is generally given by specialist occupational therapists.

In the first year the patient will need to attend the disablement service centre every two or three months for his prosthesis to be altered as the residual limb changes in shape and size. The prescription is reviewed as the patient becomes more expert. Once the artificial limb fits properly and is comfortable the patient needs to attend only about once a year for mechanical maintenance to be carried out or for possible updating of the prosthesis. Children with limb prostheses need to attend every three or four months throughout their growth period.

Common clinical problems

Artificial limb users may experience discomfort from excessive local pressure on the residual limb. In extreme cases this may lead to skin ulceration. Low back pain can occur if an artificial leg is too long or too short, but the pain may not be related to the prosthesis at all. Problems such as these can only be dealt with at the disablement service centre.

General care

Artificial limbs should be regularly examined for visible damage. Sockets are best cleaned with a damp soapy cloth and then dried. The foam liner of a patella tendon bearing limb should be removed from the socket and left out overnight to dry. No attempt should be made to lubricate any part of an artificial limb, as some components deteriorate on contact with oil. For a patient to walk properly shoes must fit his artificial foot firmly.

Artificial limbs are basically simple mechanical devices; they are most reliable, particularly considering the heavy cyclical loading a leg must bear. If a mechanical fault becomes apparent it is essential to obtain help as soon as possible from the skilled, specialist staff at the nearest disablement service centre. If someone who is not an expert attempts to alter a prosthesis there is a risk to the user; furthermore, irreparable damage may be caused to an expensive item.

The sock is an important part of the interface between the patient's skin and the prosthesis. Socks are available from the disablement service centre in a range of shapes and sizes to suit different residual limbs. Wool is the material most commonly used; it provides a resilient, moisture absorbent surface and is well tolerated by most patients. Nylon and cotton socks are available and are useful when a patient is sensitive to wool. These materials are of different thicknesses, so minor adjustments to the fit of the socket can be achieved. Socks must be washed carefully, following the written instructions given; and they should be changed regularly to avoid skin problems.

Dangers

Patients with artificial legs have delayed proprioception and impaired balance. They should therefore be made aware of the danger of tripping over low obstructions, stairs, slopes, and uneven or slippery surfaces. Knee locks, if fitted, should be used in potentially dangerous situations.

General points

If a leg has been amputated application for the mobility allowance and for a disabled car badge should be considered.

It may be necessary to adapt the patient's car. Drivers with artificial limbs should be reminded that the licensing authority must be informed of their condition.

Thought should be given to the provision of other mobility aids, such as walking frames.

Patients of working age who have had a limb amputated need advice about employment, and referral to the disablement resettlement officer may be appropriate.

Appendix

Disablement service centres (previously artificial limb and appliance centres)

England

Oak Tree Lane, Selly Oak, Birmingham B29 6JA (021 414 1661)
Elm Grove, Brighton BN2 3EX (0273 67491–6)
Government Buildings, Vassall Road, Bristol BS16 2LZ (0272 653201–3)
Hills Road, Cambridge CB2 2DB (0223 242835)
Cumberland Infirmary, Infirmary Street, Carlisle CA2 7HY (0228 29860)
Middlesbrough General Hospital, Ayrsome Green Lane, Middlesbrough, Cleveland TS5 5AZ (0642 823521)
Princess Elizabeth Orthopaedic Hospital, Wonford Road, Exeter EX2 4DU (0392 57731)
Medway Hospital, Windmill Road, Gillingham ME7 5PA (0634 811356–7)
Harold Wood Hospital, Gubbins Lane, Harold Wood, Romford RM3 0AR (040 23 74121–9)
Harehills Lane, Chapel Allerton, Leeds LS7 4EZ (0532 624791)
Knighton Street, Leicester LE2 7FB (0533 541414)
Mill Road Hospital, Liverpool L6 2AJ (051 263 7441–6, 051 263 8333)
Roehampton Lane, London SW15 5PR (01 789 6500)
Withington Hospital, Cavendish Road, Manchester M20 8LB (061 434 3311)
Freeman Road, Newcastle upon Tyne NE7 7AF (091 2856261)
Sherwood Hospital, Hucknall Road, Nottingham NG5 1PJ (0602 606026–9, 0602 603117–8)
Windmill Road, Headington, Oxford OX3 7DD (0865 63581)
St Mary's Hospital, Milton Road, Portsmouth PO3 6AD (0705 824121, 0705 829571–3)
Sharoe Green Lane North, Fulwood, Preston PR2 4US (0772 716921–4, 0772 719885)
Herries Road, Sheffield S5 7AT (0742 561571)

Wales

Prudential Building, 7 Kingsway, Cardiff, Glamorgan CF1 4LL (0222 825111)
Morriston Hospital, Heol-Maes Eglwys, Morriston, Swansea SA6 6LG (0792 795252)

Scotland

Old Infirmary Buildings, Woolmanhill, Aberdeen (0224 681818)
133 Queen Street, Broughty Ferry, Dundee (0382 730104)
Princess Margaret Rose Orthopaedic Hospital, Fairmilehead, Edinburgh 10 (031 445 4123)
Belvidere Hospital, London Road, Glasgow E1 (041 554 1855)
Mearnskirk Hospital, Newton Mearns, Glasgow (041 639 2251)
Raigmore Hospital, Inverness (0463 34151)

Northern Ireland

Musgrave Park Hospital, Stockmans Lane, Belfast BT9 7JB (0232 669501)

Useful addresses

The National Association for the Limbless Disabled, 31 The Mall, Ealing, London W5 2PX

The British Limbless Ex-Servicemens Association, Frankland Moore House, 185–187 High Road, Chadwell Heath, Essex RM6 6NA

British Amputee Sports Association, Harvey Road, Aylesbury HP21 9PP

"Reach," The Association for Children with Artificial Arms, 13 Park Terrace, Crimchard, Chard, Somerset TA20 1LA

Stomas and appliances

PAUL FINAN

The word "stoma" is derived from the Greek, meaning mouth or opening. Generally it refers to the opening constructed when the bowel has to be brought to the skin surface to convey gastrointestinal contents or urine to the exterior. The more common reasons for creating a stoma and some of the reasons for choosing between small or large bowel are listed in the box.

In the United Kingdom there are about 100 000 patients with a

---

Types of stoma and common reasons for their formation

Colostomy—Bringing a part of the large bowel to the skin surface in the treatment of
- colorectal malignancy
- inflammatory bowel disease—for example, Crohn's disease
- other inflammatory conditions of the colon—for example, diverticular disease
- traumatic diseases to the colon
- congenital and acquired neurological and anatomical abnormalities affecting normal defecation.

Ileostomy—Bringing the terminal small bowel to the skin surface in the treatment of
- inflammatory bowel disease—for example, Crohn's disease, ulcerative colitis
- temporary protection of a distal colonic anastomosis
- any trauma resulting in the excision of all the large bowel
- other causes of planned excision of the large bowel—for example, familial adenomatous polyposis coli.

Urostomy—Any opening to divert urinary drainage—most frequently an isolated ileal loop with implanted ureters—in the treatment of
- bladder carcinoma
- congenital urogenital conditions
- neuropathic bladder
- difficult urinary fistulae.

---

colostomy, 10 000 with an ileostomy, and a further 2000–3000 with a urostomy. This article reviews some of the more common physical problems encountered with stomas and related appliances and suggests ways in which these can be minimised.

Preparation for the stoma

The decision to fashion a stoma may be inevitable and indeed the operation may be carried out as an emergency; nevertheless, there is often time to prepare the patient for the procedure. Such preparation includes surgical considerations; noting physical handicaps that may severely compromise the chance of a successful independent existence; and, most importantly, consideration of the major psychological implications.

Surgical considerations—Before the operation is done it is now common practice to place an appliance on the chosen site and then encourage the patient to sit, stand, bend, and lie down. The site selected is marked before surgery. The surgical techniques are now well established. Stomas should be made away from bony landmarks, previous incisions, and areas of scarring. Moreover, they should be easy for the patient to see.

Physical considerations—Patients considered for a stoma may suffer from many disabilities, particularly if they are elderly. Some may have such poor eyesight that they cannot see well enough to change their appliance or cut holes in the flange to fit over the stoma; a metal ring cutter may help in such cases. Similarly, one can predict problems in patients with inflammatory joint disease—for example, rheumatoid arthritis—whose manual dexterity is inevitably poor. Patients in wheelchairs may be unable easily to gain access either to the stoma or the necessary toilet facilities.

Psychological considerations—The psychological implications are immense. Although patients may realise the severity of the underlying disease and thus the need for a stoma, they are nevertheless almost always shocked at seeing the stoma. They may take many months to adjust, and often never fully accept the situation.

There are feelings of anxiety; there is depression; awareness of the change in body image is strong; there are worries about family and sexual relationships. Discussion with health care personnel and perhaps an introduction at an early stage to someone who already has a stoma may help.

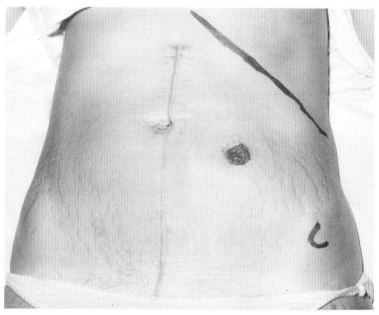

Position of permanent colostomy: away from costal margin, umbilicus, bony pelvis, and scars.

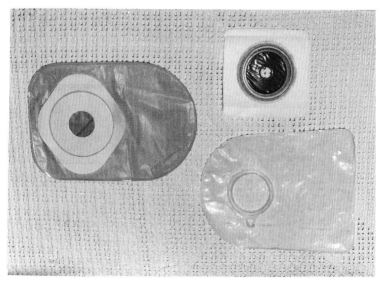

Examples of one piece *(left)* and two piece *(right)* appliances.

Types of stoma and appliances

The stoma may be fashioned from either ileum or colon and may be temporary or permanent. Fortunately many of the mechanical problems encountered are associated with the temporary stoma; these may be corrected by early re-establishment of intestinal continuity. By virtue of their site in the gastrointestinal tract, ileostomies function continuously, as do urostomies. These stomas usually drain into an appliance. There have been major improvements in the design of stoma appliances, and most patients now use disposable plastic bags. A stoma appliance consists of a bag and an adhesive flange. The flange and bag may be one piece or separate. In the two piece system the flange, once firmly fixed to the skin, may stay in place for several days and the bags may be changed at will. This system is often used in the early postoperative period: the flange can be cut precisely to cover the stoma and the patient in the early learning stage has to worry only about changing the bag, not the whole system. The disposable bags may be drainable or non-drainable. With an ileostomy or urostomy, in which the stoma functions continuously, a drainable bag is an advantage; on the other hand, most patients with colostomies prefer to use non-drainable bags.

Because the chief function of the colon is to absorb water, the more distal in the gastrointestinal system one makes a stoma the more solid the effluent and the more intermittent its action. Patients with a permanent colostomy may learn at what time of day the stoma functions and may simply wear a gauze dressing over the colostomy for most of the time. Others practise irrigation. They instil 1–1·5 litres of warm water slowly and then allow it to run out through a disposable system into the toilet. By this means the colon is kept fairly empty of faecal residue, so again an appliance is unnecessary.

Problems with the stoma

Problems may occur with (a) the stoma itself; (b) the consistency of the gastrointestinal contents; (c) the peristomal skin.

Stomas may become ischaemic immediately after the operation. This is more common in end stomas than in temporary "loop" ileostomies and colostomies. Many recover, but occasionally they have to be refashioned. Prolapse of the stoma, recognised by a sudden increase in the size of the stoma and amount protruding from the skin, is a particular problem with transverse loop colostomies and may make it almost impossible to fix the appliance. Prolapse seldom resolves spontaneously: the stoma should either be closed as soon as possible or be refashioned. Retraction of the stoma happens more with ileostomy and it may lead to severe problems with peristomal inflammation and stomal stenosis. Again, a surgical correction may be necessary, with adequate fixation of the emergent bowel.

Not only can parastomal hernias cause intermittent intestinal obstruction, they can also lead to difficulties in fitting an appliance. If such a hernia becomes a problem it is best to resite the stoma. Excessive fluid output, particularly from an ileostomy, may result in considerable depletion of water and electrolytes. Causes include recurrent active disease—for example, Crohn's disease—subacute intestinal obstruction, intraperitoneal sepsis, or a course of antibiotic therapy for an unrelated ailment. Treatment consists of rehydration, correction of the cause, and the use of drugs to slow gastrointestinal transit—for example, codeine phosphate, loperamide, or diphenoxylate hydrochloride.

Changes in stoma function are less serious but nevertheless worrying; they are often due to dietary indiscretions. Liquid stools can occur after eating green vegetables or fruit or drinking alcohol.

Excessive flatus can occur with either an ileostomy or a colostomy. But in the patient with a colostomy the flatus is accompanied by odour. Excessive flatus can be avoided by reducing foods that produce gas—for example, carbohydrates, greens, onions—and foods that produce an odour—for example, fish, eggs, cheese. A way of coping with odour is to allow the flatus to escape through a charcoal filter fitted to the appliance.

Peristomal skin

Inflammation of the peristomal skin affects up to half of all patients with ostomies at some time.

Contact dermatitis is caused by sensitivity to the appliance. It can be recognised by a distinct margin associated with the appliance and the fact that it is itchy rather than sore. Use of the new hypoallergenic materials has made the condition rarer. The more common *effluent dermatitis* can occur after prolonged contact with intestinal contents; in severe cases it can lead to desquamation and possibly secondary bacterial or fungal infection.

Initial treatment for both forms of dermatitis is the same. The skin is cleaned and then protected by a layer of Stomadhesive or Karaya gel; in severe cases steroid creams may be necessary and, if appropriate, a topical antifungal agent may be used. When the skin improves the appropriate action is to change the appliance in cases of contact dermatitis or ensure that faecal spillage does not occur on unprotected skin by having a well fitting appliance round the stoma. In these cases the advantage of the two piece system is that the flange needs to be changed less often.

Appliances

The purpose of the appliance is to collect the effluent of the stoma safely and with no leak or odour. While he is in hospital the patient will be introduced to a wide variety of appliances, but perhaps the most important step is to find one he feels comfortable with and then stay with it. In the period immediately after the operation it is usual to use a two piece system while the stoma heals and to use clear bags so that the stoma may be observed for signs of ischaemia. However, one piece systems and opaque bags may be preferable later.

Less use is now made of supporting belts; but they can give added security to patients with a urostomy when the weight of urine could cause the adhesive flange of an appliance to give way. Bag covers are useful, particularly if sweating under the plastic is a problem or a patient is worried by the "rustling" of the appliance. Secure fitting of the appliance to the skin is most often achieved with the adhesives Karaya or Stomadhesive, and if there are any irregularities of the skin contour these can be filled with Karaya gum. Odour may be controlled by using deodorant drops in the bag or by using a charcoal filter, which is either fitted to the bag or, more frequently, comes as an integral part of the appliance.

The patient will soon establish his own routine for emptying the bags. He will often keep a variety of necessary items with him, including a plastic bag for soiled bags, tissue or gauze to clean the peristomal skin, a pair of scissors, a clean appliance, and so on. The disposal of bags may be a problem. Although many authorities will collect used bags, patients often wrap them in newspaper and put them in the dustbin or burn them. They should not be flushed down the toilet as they are likely to block the drain. Most patients cut the corner of the bag, empty the contents, rinse the bag out, wrap it in a newspaper, and place it in a plastic bag.

Several companies have many years' experience with a wide range of appliances. Close cooperation with such companies is encouraged, and one often finds that the advice of their representatives is based on extensive experience. Many of them produce helpful booklets, which can be given to the patient.

Support groups

Besides a medical team and general surgical nursing staff, many centres now have special stoma care nurses (enterostomal nurses). Stoma care became an option for nurses in the 1950s; now there are more than 200 enterostomal nurses. These specialist nurses often establish stoma care clinics and may also visit patients at home. They are often available for advice at the hospital.

There are national bodies uniquely concerned with the support of patients with ileostomies, colostomies, and urostomies. One of the ways in which these organisations help is by arranging for patients to be visited before surgery. After the operation they provide much needed psychological support to those who want it.

I thank Sister D Jones for her advice in the preparation of this chapter.

Further reading

Devlin HB. *Stoma therapy review.* Coloplast Ltd, Bridge House, Orchard Lane, Huntingdon, Cambridgeshire.
Rubin GP, Devlin HB. The quality of life with a stoma. *Br J Hosp Med* 1987;**38**:300–6.
Equipment for the disabled—incontinence and stoma care. Oxfordshire Health Authority.
Gruner O-PN, Nass R, Fretheim B, Gjone E. Marital and sexual adjustments after colectomy. *Scand J Gastroenterol* 1977;**12**:193–7.
Kennedy HJ, Lee ECG, Claridge G, Truelove SC. The health of subjects living with a permanent ileostomy. *Q J Med* 1982;**203**:341–57.
Rubin GP. Aspects of stoma care in general practice. *J R Coll Gen Pract* 1986;**36**:369–70.
Burnham WR, Lennard-Jones JE, Brooke BN. Sexual problems among married ileostomates. *Gut* 1977;**18**:673–7.

Appendix

Useful addresses

Colostomy Welfare Group, 38–39 Eccleston Square, London SW1 1PB (01 828 5175)
Ileostomy Association of Great Britain and Ireland, Amblehurst House, Chobham, Woking, Surrey GU24 8PZ (09905 8277)
Urostomy Association, 8 Coniston Close, Dane Bank, Denton, Manchester M34 2EW (061 336 8818)

Explanatory booklets

Living with your ileostomy; Living with your colostomy; Living with your urostomy. Coloplast Ltd, Bridge House, Orchard Lane, Huntingdon, Cambridgeshire PE18 6QT.

Understanding colostomy; Understanding urostomy. Squibb Surgical Ltd, Squibb House, 141–149 Staines Road, Hounslow TW33 3JB.

Disabled living centres

M ANNE CHAMBERLAIN

Many diseases of the locomotor system result in loss of mobility. Many neurological diseases result in impaired manipulation of objects, diminished grip, and shortened reach. Diseases of other systems also impair function. When a person's independence in self care, ability to hold down a job, or run a household is affected technical aids may help to overcome the problem.

The exact number of technical aids on the market is unknown: there may be as many as 11 000. Certainly there are 10 200 on the database of the Disabled Living Foundation. These aids vary from an eggcup with a suction base to the sophisticated environmental controls that enable the tetraplegic patient to have some control over his environment, use the telephone, and turn on the television. How is the practitioner to decide which of these is useful to his patient?

The disabled living centre can help. There are 26 of these centres (see map). Though autonomous, they liaise with one another regularly. They may be found in hospitals or in city centres; occasionally they are in purpose built buildings, usually with wheelchair access. They all have similar aims: education and the provision of information. Each has a display of technical aids and a professional, well informed staff (mainly occupational therapists and physiotherapists). Visitors are given advice on equipment, the opportunity to try it out, and information about their disability. Centres are open during normal working hours to disabled people and their helpers as well as to professionals. Referral from a doctor is not necessary, though it does help the advisory staff if information on diagnosis and prognosis is available. For instance, it may not be appropriate to recommend installation of an expensive stair lift for someone whose life expectancy is short. However, if the patient has motor neurone disease the staff may recommend appropriate aids which can be obtained without delay. A disabled visitor asking for kitchen aids will often need a full assessment in other areas—for example, of his or her ability to take a bath or use the lavatory. The staff thus organise an appointment system with sufficient time to consider each patient's needs.

There are differences in function, size of display area, and specialist advice available. But most centres include sections on bathing, incontinence, toilet aids, low pressure beds and cushions, hoists, and incontinence aids. The nation's bill for the treatment of pressure sores is huge. It could be reduced by more widespread use of low pressure beds and cushions, which lessen the pressure on ischaemic areas. Severely disabled patients who cannot move from bed to chair often rely heavily on their carers, who may develop backache. The burdens of carers could be eased by the use of hoists and a variety of sophisticated beds. Incontinence keeps many indoors and in night-clothes. Aids for incontinence are improving and some manufacturers produce attractive clothes for the incontinent. Attractive clothes are also available for mishapened adolescents, whose confidence is shattered when they look in the mirror. A children's section, a kitchen section, and areas devoted to outdoor self propelled wheelchairs, low vision aids, communication aids, alarm systems, and environmental controls may be found in the centres.

Disabled living centres do not supply aids (Leicester being an exception). The staff recommend equipment which will alleviate the patients' problems; they also supply leaflets, costings, and details of where aids may be bought privately or obtained through health services and social services. The centres provide an excellent show-room for equipment but are entirely independent of the manu-facturers, who are usually happy to loan current items such as wheelchairs, showers, and baths. British Gas often provides a display of its adapted equipment. So does British Telecom.

Most disabled living centres organise demonstrations—for example, of alarms and call systems—and day and half day study courses on topics such as care of stroke patients, pressure relief, and leisure activities for the disabled. These demonstrations and courses are planned in response to requests from community physiotherapists, district nurses, and others. The centres also run courses for doctors but, unhappily, few seem interested in technical aids or the facilities of a centre.[1] Those who do attend are often intrigued by the equipment demonstrated. A small charge is usually made for sessions designed for professionals (many centres are only partly funded by statutory bodies and need to raise funds), but patients are not charged. In Leeds we ensure that all general practitioners in training

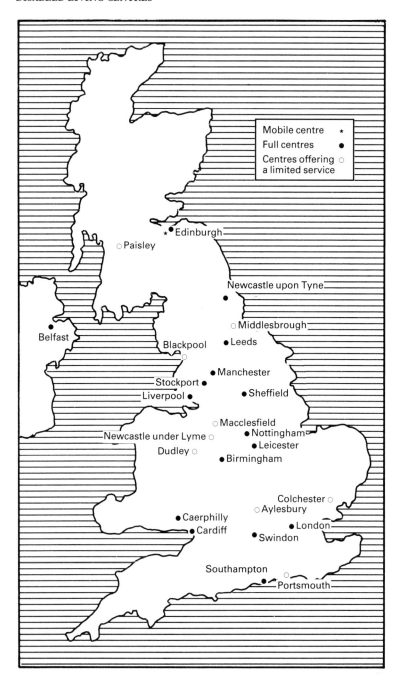

visit the centre. We have found, however, that few doctors are trained in recognising, assessing, or treating physical disability. Their use of the disabled living centre as a source of information and practical help is infrequent.

Heinz Wolff emphasised that items of equipment for the disabled should not be called "aids."[2] Certainly this word now has an unfortunate connotation. "Tools for living" is perhaps more appropriate. The able bodied use mixers, drills, and computers to do specific jobs. We must ensure that the 10% of our population who are disabled also have the basic equipment to do their work and live their lives to the full. Disabled living centres can help greatly. Why not go and see for yourself?

1 Stowe J. Disabled living centres. *J R Coll Gen Pract* 1988;**38**:306, 334, 335.
2 Wolff H. Tools for living. *Action Magazine* 1979:26-32. (National Fund for Research Into Crippling Diseases, No 26.)

Appendix

Centres offering a comprehensive service

Belfast	Disabled Living Centre Prosthetic, Orthotic and Aids Service, Musgrave Park Hospital, Stockman's Lane, Belfast BT9 7JB (0232 669501)
Birmingham	Disabled Living Centre, 260 Broad Street, Birmingham B1 2HF (021 643 0980)
Caerphilly	Resources (Aids and Equipment) Centre, Wales Council for the Disabled, Caerbragdy Industrial Estate, Bedwas Road, Caerphilly, Mid Glamorgan CF8 3SL (0222 887325–6–7)
Cardiff	The Demonstration Aids Centre, The Lodge, Rookwood Hospital, Llandaff, Cardiff, South Glamorgan CF5 2YN (0222 566281)
Edinburgh	Disabled Living Centre, Astley Ainslie Hospital, Grange Loan, Edinburgh EH9 2HL (031 447 6271)
Leeds	The William Merritt Disabled Living Centre, St Mary's Hospital, Greenhill Road, Leeds LS12 3QE (0532 793140)
Leicester	TRAIDS (Trent Region Aids, Information and Demonstration Service), 76 Clarendon Park Road, Leicester LE2 3AD (0533 700747–8)
Liverpool	Merseyside Disabled Living Centre, Youens Way, East Prescott Road, Liverpool L14 2EP (051 228 9221)

London	Disabled Living Foundation, Equipment Centre, 380–384 Harrow Road, London W9 2HU (01 289 6111)
Manchester	Disabled Living Services, Disabled Living Centre, Redbank House, 4 St Chad's Street, Cheetham, Manchester M8 8QA (061 832 3678)
Newcastle upon Tyne	Newcastle upon Tyne Council for the Disabled, The Dene Centre, Castles Farm Road, Newcastle upon Tyne NE3 1PH (091 2840480)
Nottingham	Nottingham Resource Centre for the Disabled, Lenton Business Centre, Lenton Boulevard, Nottingham NG7 2BY (0602 420391)
Sheffield	Sheffield Independent Living Centre, 108 The Moor, Sheffield S1 4DP (0742 737025)
Southampton	Southampton Aid and Equipment Centre, Southampton General Hospital, Tremona Road, Southampton SO9 4XY (0703 777222)
Stockport	Disabled Living Centre, Stockport Area Health Authority, St Thomas's Hospital, Shawheath, Stockport SK3 8BL (061 419 4476)
Swindon	The Swindon Centre for Disabled Living, The Hawthorn Centre, Cricklade Road, Swindon, Wiltshire SN2 1AF (0793 643966)

Centres offering a limited service

Aylesbury	Dial and Smile (South Corridor), Stoke Mandeville Hospital, Mandeville Road, Aylesbury, Buckinghamshire HP21 8AL (0296 84111)
Blackpool	Disabled Living Centre, 8 Queen Street, Blackpool, Lancashire FY1 1PD (0253 21084)
Colchester	Disabled Living Centre, OT Department, Colchester General Hospital, Colchester, Essex CO4 5JL (0206 853535)
Dudley	Dudley Disabled Living Centre, 1 St Giles Street, Netherton, Dudley DY2 0PR (0384 237034)
Huddersfield	Disabled Living Centre, Silver Court, Silver Street, Huddersfield HD5 9AG (0484 518809)
Macclesfield	Centre for Disabled Living, Macclesfield District General Hospital, Macclesfield, Cheshire SK10 3BL (0625 21000)
Middlesbrough	Department of Rehabilitation, Middlesbrough General Hospital, Ayresome Green Lane, Middlesbrough, Cleveland TS5 5AZ (0642 813133)
Newcastle under Lyme	Independent Living Centre (The Arts Centre), Brampton Park, Newcastle under Lyme, Staffordshire ST5 0QP (0782 634949)
Paisley	Disability Centre for Independent Living, Community Services Centre, Queen Street, Paisley, Scotland (041 887 0597)

Portsmouth   Disabled Living Centre, Prince Albert Road, Eastney, Portsmouth PO4 9HR (0705 737174)

Mobile advice centre

Scottish Council on Disability, Princess House, 5 Shandwick Place, Edinburgh EH2 4RG (031 229 8632)

Provision of aids

GRAHAM P MULLEY

Consider a patient who is about to leave hospital. Suppose that the consultant failed to prescribe digoxin for his rapid atrial fibrillation or diuretics for heart failure. The patient has, however, been given appropriate medication for his other conditions; but he has been told that tablets are to be obtained from one source and capsules from another, that ointment comes from a third source, and inhalers from a fourth. He also needs a bottle of medicine, but he is not told where to get it. No one shows him how to use the inhaler, or troubles to find out whether he understands how his tablets should be taken. Without his medication his general condition will deteriorate. Yet a week or two may elapse before he gets most of his medicaments; and some items may not materialise until three months later.

Such a situation would be intolerable. Fortunately, failure to consider drug therapy, ensure compliance, and provide medication promptly are recognised as bad practice; and our traditional medical training has equipped us with a sound pharmacological basis for treating many illnesses. But unfortunately our training does not encourage us to think of aids, appliances, and adaptations that can help overcome or compensate for disability. The provision of aids would be improved by a greater awareness by professionals and the general public, a simpler and more efficient system of supplying aids, and better education of patients and families in their use.

Will this patient benefit from an aid or appliance?

We prescribe Levodopa for parkinsonism; but we do not always consider whether high seat chairs, raised toilet seats, bath aids, and devices to facilitate turning in bed might improve patients' mobility and thus help them to maintain their independence. We prescribe analgesics for arthritis but often fail to recommend mobility aids, which can reduce pain in weight bearing joints. Sometimes we fail to realise that a stroke patient needs a commode if he is no longer able to walk upstairs to the toilet. Only half the incontinent elderly people living at home are provided with pads or other continence aids.

It is always useful to ask disabled patients to describe difficulties they may experience during a typical day. You can then recommend aids to help with those activities that present problems. Doctors and other health workers can obtain useful advice on aids and appliances from occupational therapists. Some other sources of information are listed in the appendix.

If, in future, there were to be high street shops specialising in aids for the disabled both patients and their families would become more aware of the range of aids available. Wolff[1] envisages centres—for example, "granny care" shops—where skilled staff would provide informed, objective advice on the most suitable aid. At present aids bought privately are not always appropriate to the patient's needs—especially walking sticks, commodes, chairs, and feeding aids.

Improving the supply of aids

The provision of aids is complex and fragmented. Wheelchairs are obtained from the Department of Health and Social Security through disablement service centres, but ramps to facilitate the movement of wheelchairs in and out of the house are provided by local authority housing departments, sometimes after a long delay. Walking aids are available from physiotherapists and from social services; social services also supply aids for daily living, such as bathing and toilet aids. There is an overlap in the provision of aids by social services and health authorities, the pattern varying from district to district. Special footwear, corsets, and braces can only be obtained through the hospital service when a consultant has given his approval. Younger disabled people may obtain aids to employment from the Manpower Services Commission on the recommendation of the disablement resettlement officer.

The storage of individual aids by different agencies on separate sites can mean that a community nurse wishing to obtain a commode for a patient may waste much time contacting the community nursing depot, hospital stores, social services, and the Red Cross.[2] Even then, she may be unable to find the right commode for her patient.

Given the complexity of the system it is not surprising that the provision of aids is often slow and unsatisfactory. The distress caused by delays of a month or more before incontinence pads or commodes could be obtained for dying patients has been reported. So have the unacceptable delays in the provision of bath aids for disabled patients discharged from hospital. One survey revealed that 40% of those needing wheelchairs had to wait over a month. In Edinburgh, where 80% of aids were provided within a month to stroke victims, a wait of over six months for stair rails or ramps meant that some patients were prevented from going outside unaided.

A sensible solution would be for each district general hospital to have a central equipment centre such as the one at Salisbury.[2] These could house the whole range of aids, which would be loaned to patients in or about to leave hospital as well as to the disabled living at home. The artificial demarcations between health and social services aids would be eased and communications between these agencies improved; costs could be reduced by bulk buying; the streamlined provision of equipment would allow more efficient use of health workers' time; the prompt provision of aids would reduce distress to patients and carers and ensure better use of equipment. These centres would be run by occupational therapists, who would also provide an advice and information service and stimulate research in the design, provision, and use of aids.

Ensuring that aids are used and useful

In a study of 500 elderly and disabled people in receipt of aids and appliances, it was found that one third of feeding aids and one fifth of bath aids and toilet aids had never been used. At the time of the assessment 50% of all aids were not in use. There is little point in buying, storing, and delivering aids if they are not going to benefit the patient. There are several reasons why aids are not used:

(1) The aid may be poorly designed, being too complicated, uncomfortable, unattractive, socially unacceptable—people usually prefer ordinary utensils to modified eating and drinking aids—or ineffective.

(2) The aid may be ill fitting or unsafe; common examples are loose or slippery bath rails and mats, and worn or defective walking aids.

(3) The patient and family may have received little or no instruction in the use of aids. In one survey only 14% of disabled people had been given the chance to try a raised toilet seat before provision. Of 750 disabled adults, only half received instructions when the aid was issued and very few received further education.

(4) The patient's condition may have improved (a quarter of aids

are provided to those whose disability is temporary) or deteriorated. The changing need for aids by patients with progressive disorders such as motor neurone disease and parkinsonism should be regularly reviewed by the community occupational therapist.

(5) The patient may prefer personal help to gadgets: increased social contact may be more important than the greater independence provided by technical aids.

Retrieval

In a study of common aids to daily living provided by social services in a London borough, 15% of aids were unused and retained by the patient. In Edinburgh, only 10% of stroke patients returned unused aids. Twenty two per cent of bath and toilet aids given to patients after hip replacement remained unused at home after six months.

If aids are retrieved, cleaned, and repaired they can be used for other patients. There are several ways of achieving this:

- *Labelling*—If the address and telephone number is on the equipment the patient will be reminded that the aid is on loan and may be more likely to return it.
- *Deposits*—The cost of accounting and the financial plight of many disabled and elderly people may make this proposal unrealistic.
- *Publicity campaigns*—Posters in surgeries and announcements on local radio may encourage people to return unused aids.
- *Follow up letters*—Care must be taken that these do not upset patients and relatives, who may fear that much needed aids are going to be taken from them. Letters may be mistakenly sent to people who have returned their aids, or to those who have died.
- *Retrieval by health professionals*—The development of a single central store might allow return of aids by doctors, nurses, therapists, social workers, and others seeing patients at home.

Ensuring that aids are returned does not always make financial sense: the cost of transport, inspection, and correction of faults make it illogical to recycle some cheaper aids. Further studies of the cost effectiveness of retrieval and reutilisation are needed before this practice is widely adopted.

1 Wolff HS. Tools for living: a blueprint for a major new industry. In: Bray J, Wright S, eds. *The use of technology in the care of the elderly and disabled. Tools for living.* London: Pinter, 1980:130–6.
2 Robertson JC, Haines JR. A community/hospital home aids and loan scheme (based on a rehabilitation demonstration centre). *Hlth Trends* 1978;**10**:15–6.

Recommended reading

Darnbrough A, Kinrade D. *Directory for disabled people*, 4th edn. Cambridge: Woodhead-Faulkner Ltd, 1985, 358. (Contains a section on the provision and availability of aids.)

Equipment for the Disabled. A series of excellent reference books on aids and appliances obtainable from Mary Marlborough Lodge, Nuffield Orthopaedic Centre, Headington, Oxford OX3 7LD.

DHSS Leaflet HB1 (S). *Help for handicapped people in Scotland.*

DHSS Leaflet HB2. *Aids for the disabled.*

(DHSS leaflets are available from local DHSS offices or from DHSS Leaflets Unit, PO Box 21, Stanmore, Middlesex HA7 1AY.)

Appendix

Where to get information on aids and appliances

United Kingdom

Disabled Living Foundation, 380–384 Harrow Road, London W9 2HU (01 289 6111)

Scottish Council on Disability, Princes House, 5 Shandwick Place, Edinburgh EH2 4RG (031 229 8632)

Northern Ireland Information Service for Disabled People, 2 Arndale Avenue, Belfast BT7 3JH (0232 640011)

These organisations provide information, lists, and bulletins on a wide range of aids and appliances as well as an advisory service for patients, families, and professionals.

The Royal Association for Disability and Rehabilitation (RADAR), 25 Mortimer Street, London W1N 8AB (01 637 5400). It provides a useful list of publications for the disabled.

Disabled living centres (see appendix to previous chapter).

Overseas

International Disability Education and Awareness, 16 Bath Street, Frome, Somerset BA11 1DN (0373 67006)

Appropriate Health Resources and Technologies Action Group Ltd (AHRTAG), 85 Marylebone High Street, London W1M 3DE (01 486 4175)

These organisations produce literature on aids and appliances for disabled people who live in developing countries.

Index